The Runner

Guest Editor

ROBERT P. WILDER, MD, FACSM

CLINICS IN SPORTS MEDICINE

www.sportsmed.theclinics.com

Consulting Editor
MARK D. MILLER, MD

July 2010 • Volume 29 • Number 3

SAUNDERS an imprint of ELSEVIER, Inc.

W.B. SAUNDERS COMPANY

A Division of Elsevier Inc.

1600 John F. Kennedy Blvd. ● Suite 1800 ● Philadelphia, Pennsylvania 19103

http://www.theclinics.com

CLINICS IN SPORTS MEDICINE Volume 29, Number 3
July 2010 ISSN 0278-5919, ISBN-13: 978-1-4377-2497-4

Editor: Ruth Malwitz
Developmental Editor: Donald Mumford

Clinics in Sports Medicine (ISSN 0278-5919) is published quarterly by Elsevier Inc., 360 Park Avenue South, New York, NY 10010-1710. Months of issue are January, April, July, and October. Business and Editorial Offices: 1600 John F. Kennedy Blvd., Ste. 1800, Philadelphia, PA 19103-2899. Customer Service Office: 3251 Riverport Lane, Maryland Heights, MO 63043. Periodicals postage paid at New York, NY and additional mailing offices. Subscription prices are $278.00 per year (US individuals), $424.00 per year (US institutions), $140.00 per year (US students), $315.00 per year (Canadian individuals), $512.00 per year (Canadian institutions), $195.00 (Canadian students), $382.00 per year (foreign individuals), $512.00 per year (foreign institutions), and $195.00 per year (foreign students). Foreign air speed delivery is included in all *Clinics* subscription prices. All prices are subject to change without notice. **POSTMASTER:** Send address changes to *Clinics in Sports Medicine*, Elsevier Health Sciences Division, Subscription Customer Service, 3251 Riverport Lane, Maryland Heights, MO 63043. Customer Service (orders, claims, online, change of address): Elsevier Health Sciences Division, Subscription Customer Service, 3251 Riverport Lane, Maryland Heights, MO 63043. Tel: 1-800-654-2452 (U.S. and Canada); 314-447-8871 (outside U.S. and Canada). Fax: 314-447-8029. E-mail: journalscustomerservice-usa@elsevier.com (for print support); journalsonlinesupport-usa@elsevier.com (for online support).

Reprints. For copies of 100 or more of articles in this publication, please contact the Commercial Reprints Department, Elsevier Inc., 360 Park Avenue South, New York, NY 10010-1710. Tel.: 212-633-3812; Fax: 212-462-1935; E-mail: reprints@elsevier.com.

Clinics in Sports Medicine is covered in *MEDLINE/PubMed (Index Medicus) Current Contents/Clinical Medicine, Excerpta Medica,* and *ISI/Biomed.*

Printed in the United States of America.

Contributors

CONSULTING EDITOR

MARK D. MILLER, MD
S. Ward Casscells Professor of Orthopaedic Surgery, University of Virginia, Charlottesville, Virginia; Team Physician, James Madison University, Harrisonburg, Virginia

GUEST EDITOR

ROBERT P. WILDER, MD, FACSM
Harrison Distinguished Associate Professor, Chair, Department of Physical Medicine and Rehabilitation, The University of Virginia; Director, the Runner's Clinic at UVa; Team Physician, UVa Athletics; Team Physician, Ragged Mountain Racing, Charlottesville, Virginia

AUTHORS

JAMES BEAZELL, PT, DPT, OCS, ATC
Clinical Coordinator, University of Virginia–HealthSouth Physical Therapy, Charlottesville, Virginia

MARC A. CHILDRESS, MD
Department of Family and Sports Medicine, DeWitt Army Community Hospital, Fort Belvoir, Virginia

HERVÉ COLLADO, MD
Department of Medicine & Rehabilitation and Sport Medicine, University Hospital la Timone, Boulevard Jean Moulin, Marseille, France; Division of Physical Medicine and Rehabilitation, Stanford University School of Medicine; Department of Orthopaedic Surgery, Physical Medicine and Rehabilitation and Sports Medicine, Stanford University School of Medicine, Stanford, California

DANIEL COLONNO, MD
Department of Rehabilitation Medicine, University of Washington, Seattle, Washington

JAY DICHARRY, MPT
Director, The Center for Endurance Sport, Department of Physical Medicine and Rehabilitation, The University of Virginia, Charlottesville, Virginia

JONATHAN T. FINNOFF, DO
Assistant Professor, Department of Physical Medicine and Rehabilitation, Mayo Clinic Sports Medicine Center, Mayo Clinic, Rochester, Minnesota

MICHAEL FREDERICSON, MD
Professor, Orthopaedics & Sports Medicine; Director, Physical Medicine and Rehabilitation Sports Medicine Service; Team Physician, Stanford Cross-Country & Track, Stanford University School of Medicine, Stanford Center for Medicine, Redwood City, California

PAMELA A. HANSEN, MD
Assistant Professor, Division of Physical Medicine and Rehabilitation, University of Utah
Orthopaedic Center, Salt Lake City, Utah

MARK A. HARRAST, MD
Medical Director, Seattle Marathon; Clinical Associate of Professor of Rehabilitation
Medicine, Orthopaedics and Sports Medicine, University of Washington, UW Medicine
Sports and Spine, Seattle, Washington

ANNE Z. HOCH, DO
Professor, Director, Women's Sports Medicine Program, Department of Orthopaedic
Surgery, Sports Medicine Center, Medical College of Wisconsin, Milwaukee, Wisconsin

JEFFREY JENKINS, MD
Associate Professor, Department of Physical Medicine and Rehabilitation, University
of Virginia, Charlottesville, Virginia

BENJAMIN D. LEVINE, MD
S. Finley Ewing Chair for Wellness, Institute for Exercise and Environmental Medicine,
Presbyterian Hospital, University of Texas Southwestern Medical Center, Dallas, Texas

STACY L. LYNCH, MD
Fellow, Department of Orthopaedic Surgery, Sports Medicine Center, Medical College
of Wisconsin, Milwaukee, Wisconsin

ERIC MAGRUM, PT
Senior Physical Therapist, UVa Health South Physical Therapy, Charlottesville, Virginia

FRANCIS G. O'CONNOR, MD, MPH
Department of Military and Emergency Medicine, Consortium for Health and Military
Performance, Uniformed Services University of the Health Sciences, Bethesda, Maryland

EVAN PECK, MD
Sports Medicine Fellow, Department of Physical Medicine and Rehabilitation, Mayo Clinic
Sports Medicine Center, Mayo Clinic, Rochester, Minnesota

CRAIG K. SETO, MD
Associate Professor of Family Medicine, Director of Sports Medicine, Assistant
Residency Director, Department of Family Medicine, University of Virginia Health System,
Charlottesville, Virginia

JAY SMITH, MD
Professor, Department of Physical Medicine and Rehabilitation, Mayo Clinic Sports
Medicine Center, Mayo Clinic, Rochester, Minnesota

IAN L. SOLARI, MD
Family Medicine Resident, Department of Family Medicine, University of Virginia Health
System, Charlottesville, Virginia

SIOBHAN M. STATUTA, MD
Chief Resident, Department of Family Medicine, University of Virginia Health System,
Charlottesville, Virginia

ROBERT P. WILDER, MD, FACSM
Harrison Distinguished Associate Professor, Chair, Department of Physical Medicine and Rehabilitation, The University of Virginia; Director, the Runner's Clinic at UVa; Team Physician, UVa Athletics; Team Physician, Ragged Mountain Racing, Charlottesville, Virginia

STUART E. WILLICK, MD, FACSM
Associate Professor, Division of Physical Medicine and Rehabilitation, University of Utah Orthopaedic Center, Salt Lake City, Utah

Contents

> The evaluation of the injured runner emphasizes the identification of intrinsic and extrinsic risk factors in addition to establishing injury-specific diagnosis. The history emphasizes identification of contributory changes in training regimen or technique. The physical examination includes a biomechanical and functional screening to identify related imbalances in posture, alignment, strength, flexibility, and lower quarter stability. Each runner is also observed walking and running because running is a dynamic activity, and subtle abnormalities not evident during static or open chain examination may become evident upon functional and dynamic evaluation. This comprehensive, running-specific approach to diagnosis assists the clinician in developing optimum rehabilitation programs.

> Dynamic gait evaluation allows examination of the intrinsic and extrinsic factors affecting an individual's ability to walk or run. This article identifies the gait cycle so that common terminology can be used to discuss and compare walking and running. The range of motion, or kinematics, used during gait can be seen subjectively in the hallway of the clinic but can be further objectified in a motion analysis laboratory. Kinetics, or the forces that cause the body to move, are collected in a laboratory environment. Understanding the internal and external forces acting on the body, the mobility they produce at the joints, and the corresponding effect on biomechanics helps identify sources of dysfunction. A discussion on economy highlights factors affecting the ability to move with a given amount of energy cost.

> Flexibility training, commonly referred to as stretching, has become a standard part of athletic training for nearly all sports. Athletes almost universally engage in some form of flexibility training because of the perception that it prevents injury and may enhance sports performance. With specific regard to running, controversy has arisen regarding these proposed benefits of stretching. In this article, the authors seek to define

flexibility training and evaluate the evidence for its clinical benefit. They also describe the components of a general lower quarter flexibility program that they encourage their patients to follow at the University of Virginia Runner's Clinic.

Patellofemoral pain (PFP) syndrome is a frequently encountered overuse disorder that involves the patellofemoral region and often presents as anterior knee pain. PFP can be difficult to diagnose. Not only do the etiology, diagnosis, and treatment remain challenging, but the terminology used to describe PFP is used inconsistently and can be confusing. Patellofemoral pain syndrome (PFPS) seems to be multifactorial, resulting from a complex interaction among intrinsic anatomic and external training factors. Although clinicians frequently make the diagnosis of PFPS, no consensus exists about its etiology or the factors most responsible for causing pain. This article discusses the pathophysiology, diagnosis, and management of PFP.

Running has many beneficial effects, including cardiovascular and skeletal health. Poor training technique and a variety of risk factors may predispose runners to lower-limb overuse injuries affecting muscle, tendon, and bone. Injuries to the bone include stress reactions to full-fledged stress fractures. This article is designed to provide an understanding of the general concepts involving bone strain, risk factor assessment, and evaluation and treatment strategies for the runner with a stress fracture. The second half of the article presents more detail regarding each specific fracture seen in runners. The ultimate goal of this article is to provide the basics regarding stress fractures in runners from pathophysiology and general guidelines of evaluation and treatment and provide a quick reference regarding the details of each specific fracture encountered in clinical practice.

The overall health benefits of cardiovascular exercise, such as running, are well established. However, it is also well established that in certain circumstances running can lead to overload injuries of muscle, tendon, and bone. In contrast, it has not been established that running leads to degeneration of articular cartilage, which is the hallmark of osteoarthritis. This article reviews the available literature on the association between running and osteoarthritis, with a focus on clinical epidemiologic studies. The preponderance of clinical reports refutes an association between running and osteoarthritis.

Chronic exertional compartment syndrome should be considered in any runner experiencing exertional leg pain. Runners typically describe a tight,

cramping ache over the involved compartment that commences at a reproducible point in the run and resolves with rest. Diagnosis should include
a careful history and physical examination as well as documentation
with intramuscular compartment pressure monitoring. Milder cases will resolve with activity modification and conservative care. More severe cases
or those failing conservative care are referred for fasciotomy.

Neuropathies in Runners 437

Evan Peck, Jonathan T. Finnoff, and Jay Smith

Nerve entrapment represents an uncommon but important cause of lower
limb pain among runners. This article reviews the diagnosis and management of several nerve entrapment syndromes that may be encountered
among runners, but clinicians must be aware that any peripheral nerve
may be affected. Successful diagnosis and management are predicated
on several underlying principles: (1) maintain a high index of suspicion
for neurologic syndromes, (2) recognize common presentations of neuropathic pain, (3) perform a meticulous physical examination, including postexercise examination when necessary, (4) consider a broad differential
diagnosis (neurologic and nonneurologic), (5) use diagnostic testing appropriately, and (6) make rational clinical decisions, including referral for
second opinion when indicated. A thorough knowledge of neuroanatomy
and running biomechanics allows the clinician to successfully apply these
principles to almost all clinical scenarios.

**Exertional Collapse in the Runner: Evaluation and Management in Fieldside
and Office-Based Settings** 459

Marc A. Childress, Francis G. O'Connor, and Benjamin D. Levine

Exertional collapse is a commonly encountered phenomenon among
runners, particularly in the setting of long distances and extreme
environments. Although exertional collapse is generally a benign event occurring in an exhausted finisher at race completion, the multifactorial nature of this disorder creates a broad differential diagnosis. The ability of
the sports provider to appropriately recognize and treat these various potential concerns is critical, because collapse may represent several life-
threatening conditions. It is especially challenging to determine the appropriate course of evaluation and management of collapse in the context of
a mass participation event. This article presents a discussion of the etiology and pathophysiology of collapse as well as strategies for the effective
assessment and treatment of collapsed runners, whether in the fieldside
setting or in an outpatient office-based environment.

The Female Runner: Gender Specifics 477

Stacy L. Lynch and Anne Z. Hoch

There has been a tremendous increase in the number of female runners
of all ages and abilities in the past 35 years. Women who participate in
running and sports are generally healthier and have higher self-esteem.

However, unique medical and orthopedic issues exist for the female runner. This article reviews the history of women in sports, physiologic and biomechanic differences between genders, the pregnant runner, knee osteoarthritis, an update on the female athlete triad and the relationship between amenorrhea and endothelial dysfunction associated with athletics.

As more children have become involved in athletic activities and running, there has been a significant increase in overuse injuries. The young athlete with open growth plates is vulnerable to unique overuse injuries involving the apophyses, articular cartilage, and growth plate. The physician caring for these young athletes needs to be aware of these conditions to diagnose and treat them appropriately. Physicians should also be aware of the risk of overtraining and overuse injury in athletes participating in year-round sports and competition. Current guidelines for overuse injury prevention in young athletes are primarily based on consensus and expert opinion. Further research is needed to provide evidence-based guidelines for overuse injury prevention in young athletes and runners.

THE CLINICS ARE NOW AVAILABLE ONLINE!

Access your subscription at:
www.theclinics.com

Foreword
The Runner

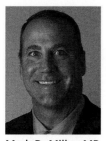

Mark D. Miller, MD
Consulting Editor

I am happy to introduce another great edition of *Clinics in Sports Medicine*. This issue focuses on the runner. Runners come in all shapes and sizes and all levels of competition, but they all seem to share the same intensity for their sport. If you are like me, you simply cannot get by with telling your patients that if it hurts, quit running. That is why I am so happy that Dr Wilder heads a premier Runner's Clinic at our institution. I have asked him to share his expertise with our readership as a guest editor for this edition; needless to say, he has done a remarkable job!

This issue begins with the basics—epidemiology, biomechanics, evaluation, and so forth; includes all of the sometimes difficult clinical entities (osteoarthritis, patellofemoral syndrome, stress fractures, and neuropathies); addresses some important considerations (collapse and flexibility); and also considers special populations (female and pediatric runners). Put it all together and you have the prefect treatise for evaluating and treating the running athlete. But do not let me run on with this Foreword any more...let us get started!

Mark D. Miller, MD
Department of Orthopaedic Surgery
University of Virginia
400 Ray C. Hunt Drive, Suite 330
Charlottesville, VA 22908-0159, USA

E-mail address:
mdm3p@virginia.edu

Clin Sports Med 29 (2010) xiii
doi:10.1016/j.csm.2010.03.011
0278-5919/10/$ – see front matter © 2010 Elsevier Inc. All rights reserved.

Preface
The Runner

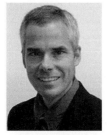

Robert P. Wilder, MD
Guest Editor

An estimated 37 million Americans run for exercise. This represents a significant increase from the 30 million Americans running at the end of the running boom of the 1980s. Some of this increase has been attributed to a greater awareness of the health benefits of exercise and, importantly, a greater number of women runners. In 1980, women accounted for 10% of participants in marathons. In 2005, 40% of all marathoners were women. Although many of these participants do so primarily for recreation and fitness, data support a resurgence of competitive participants as well. As of the writing of this preface, a total of 26 US runners have eclipsed the 4-minute mile barrier during this indoor track season alone!

Clinicians are called on to meet the increasing demands to keep runners running (and running safely) from childhood through the senior years. This issue of *Clinics in Sports Medicine* will help health care practitioners meet the specific needs of the running athlete. A comprehensive running-specific history and physical examination, and when indicated, detailed kinetic and kinematic analysis will assist the clinician in making the most specific diagnosis as well as identifying contributing factors throughout the kinetic chain. Detail is provided regarding the management of common running injuries, including patellofemoral syndrome, stress fractures, compartment syndrome, and neuropathies in runners. Special topics including management of exercise-associated collapse and the runner with osteoarthritis are developed. Special considerations for pediatric and female runners are presented. Finally, a comprehensive review of flexibility will assist the clinician in counseling runners regarding this important adjunct to cardiovascular fitness.

Clin Sports Med 29 (2010) xv–xvi
doi:10.1016/j.csm.2010.03.010
0278-5919/10/$ – see front matter © 2010 Elsevier Inc. All rights reserved.

sportsmed.theclinics.com

I would like to thank Mark Miller, MD for his vote of confidence in me to assist with this issue and for the clinical expertise he has extended to so many of my patients. I thank also the authors, all experts in running medicine, for contributing to this issue.
See you on the roads!

Robert P. Wilder, MD
Department of Physical Medicine and Rehabilitation
University of Virginia
545 Ray C. Hunt Drive #240
Charlottesville, VA 22901, USA

E-mail address:
rpw4n@virginia.edu

Evaluation of the Injured Runner

Eric Magrum, PT[a], Robert P. Wilder, MD[b],*

KEYWORDS

• Pronation • Supination • Flexibility • Patella

EXAMINATION OF THE RUNNER

Two guiding principles assist in identifying risk factors for the injured runner.[1–4] Leadbetter's principle of transition seeks to identify extrinsic risk factors[5] and states that injury is most likely to occur when the athlete experiences a change in mode or use of the involved part. Most running injuries occur when the athlete has a specific change in training, such as a change in running volume, intensity, or equipment. Accordingly, the history carefully searches to identify the change or transition.

Macintyre's principle of "victim and culprits" underscores the importance of the biomechanical and functional examination.[6] The presenting injury represents the "victim," which has occurred as a result of an inability to compensate for a primary dysfunction at another site, the "culprit." The entire kinetic chain must be examined to rule out asymptomatic injury or dysfunction. For example, the "malicious malalignment syndrome" (femoral anteversion, knee valgus with increased Q angle, external tibia torsion, heel valgus, and pronation) can, with faulty training techniques, contribute to injury.[7]

History

In addition to the standard medical history, a detailed analysis must be made of premorbid and current running history. Useful information includes weekly mileage, length of long run, pace, the number of pairs and types of running shoes worn, frequency of hill work and interval training, running surfaces, and review of flexibility, strength, warm-up exercises, and amount of cross-training activities.

Because overuse injuries are often asymptomatic in their origin, the history well before the symptoms first appeared must be inquired after. Were there antecedent changes in training routines, running shoes, or surfaces? When during running does the pain occur? Does the pain only occur with up or down hill, after a certain distance, or only when running on a particular surface? Does the pain occur during and after

[a] UVa Health South Physical Therapy, 545 Ray C. Hunt #240, Charlottesville, VA, USA
[b] Department of PM&R, University of Virginia, 545 Ray C. Hunt #240, Charlottesville, VA 22901, USA
* Corresponding author.
E-mail address: rpw4n@virginia.edu

Clin Sports Med 29 (2010) 331–345
doi:10.1016/j.csm.2010.03.009
0278-5919/10/$ – see front matter © 2010 Elsevier Inc. All rights reserved.

running? Is there any initial improvement with a period of warm-up? Self-treatments, prior medical treatments, and previous diagnostic tests should be reviewed. Finally, the health care provider should always ask the runner what he or she believes the problem to be.

Examination

Examination of the injured runner includes a sequential biomechanical screening, site-specific examination, functional screening, gait analysis, shoe wear assessment, and appropriate ancillary tests.[4,7–9]

Biomechanical Assessment

Standing

The examination of the runner begins in the standing position on an uncarpeted surface. The athlete should be in running shorts, without shirt, shoes, or socks on. The female athlete should be in an appropriate sports bra or gown. The examiner should have adequate space to step back to assess the athlete's posture. Posture is assessed by having the athlete face the examiner, face sideways, and stand with the back to the examiner. The physician should start by observing the general contour of the spine, noting abnormal curvature, shoulder or pelvic tilt, flank creases, or prominent scapula, which may suggest scoliosis. The athlete is observed bending forward and sideways, and any spinal deformities or segmental dysfunction noted. Having the athlete bend forward also allows the examiner the opportunity to assess lumbopelvic rhythm. The normal lumbar lordosis should reverse with forward flexion.

The examiner then screens the athlete for leg length discrepancies. The examiner palpates the iliac crests and anterior and posterior superior iliac spines, and notes any asymmetries. Asymmetries can represent functional or anatomic leg length discrepancies. Functional leg length discrepancies imply that the actual leg lengths are equal. Functional differences may be related to varying degrees of foot pronation or sacroiliac (SI), pelvic, or hip dysfunction. Anatomic leg length discrepancies imply that one leg is actually shorter than the other.

Sacroiliac joint function is assessed by the SI fixation and flexion tests.[10] With the SI fixation test the inferior slope of the posterior superior iliac spine and the medial spinous process of S2 are identified with the thumbs bilaterally. The patient is then asked to flex the hip. With the SI flexion test, the patient bends forward with the examiner's thumbs on the posterior superior iliac spines bilaterally. Normally the examiner's thumb swings downward and lateral. A positive test (indicating SI dysfunction) occurs when the examiner's thumb swings upward or does not move relative to the other side.

Alignment of the lower leg is assessed by sequentially observing the knees, lower legs, and feet. The knees are observed for genu valgum, varum, or recurvatum. Genu varum is not uncommon in men, with 5° representing the upper limit of normal. Genu valgum is not uncommon in women, with 5° again representing the upper limit of normal. Patellar position is noted. Normally in the standing position the patella faces directly forward; "squinting" or excessively laterally displaced patella may predispose to patellofemoral syndrome.

In the standing position, most feet can be identified as cavus, neutral, or pronated. The cavus foot is highly arched and rigid, with calcaneal inversion. The pronated foot is flexible with little to no arch being present.

The lower extremity is then examined in the subtalar neutral position. In the standing position, the foot is placed in neutral position by placing the talonavicular joint in a position of congruency. Talonavicular congruency is obtained by having the examiner place the thumb just distal to the medial malleolus at the talonavicular joint, with the middle finger just distal to the tibiofibular syndesmosis. The foot is then moved into pronation, in which position the thumb will appreciate a bulge from the talus. When the foot is supinated, the middle finger will appreciate a bulge from the talus. Talonavicular congruency, or subtalar neutral position, is appreciated when the talus is felt equally by both the thumb and the middle finger. From this position the examiner can determine the neutral tibia stance by bisecting the posterior lower one-third of the tibia, and measuring this angle with the sagittal perpendicular. Normal individuals in neutral stance will have 0° to 4° of tibia varus. The navicular drop can then be measured by having the runner relax the feet from the neutral position. The amount of movement of the navicular toward the floor is termed the navicular drop. A drop of up to 1 cm is considered normal. A drop of greater than 1.5 cm is abnormal and may indicate a heightened need for motion control, through stability exercise, shoes, or corrective orthoses.

Lower extremity flexibility and strength are then screened. Facing away from the examiner, the athlete stands up on the toes, allowing assessment of plantar flexor strength, tibialis posterior function, and rear foot motion. Normally the calcaneus swings into inversion, demonstrating normal posterior tibialis function and adequate subtalar motion. From the lateral position the examiner observes the patient flex at the knees without lifting the heels from the floor, assessing dorsiflexion motion and functional gastrocsoleus flexibility. The normal running gait requires 10° to 15° of ankle dorsiflexion.

Sitting

The athlete sits on the end of the examination table with the knees hanging over the table in 90° of flexion, allowing the examiner to reassess pelvis position and leg length and initiate an examination of the knee, including the patellofemoral joint.

Leg length discrepancies that are detected on the standing examination are further evaluated in the sitting position. Abnormalities or obliquities detected by palpating the iliac crests and/or posterior superior iliac spines are rechecked in the sitting position. If the aforementioned become level in the sitting position, a discrepancy in the leg length should be suspected. If the asymmetry persists, dysfunction of the hip, SI joint, and/or spine should be suspected.

Patellar position and tracking are assessed. In the normal individual, the patella should face directly forward when the knees are flexed 90°. Patella alta may exist if the patellae are oriented obliquely toward the ceiling. The tubercle-sulcus angle is calculated by first constructing an imaginary line through the medial and lateral epicondyles of the femur. Then a perpendicular to this line is drawn through the center of the patella. The sulcus angle is then determined by measuring the angle between this vertical line and a line drawn from the center of the patella to the center of the tibial tubercle. The normal angle is less than 8° in women and 5° in men.

The examiner observes active patellar tracking. With normal active extension the patella tracks straight superior or lateral to superior in a 1:1 ratio. The examiner than places a hand over the patella and palpates for crepitus, noting the severity as well as the point of occurrence during knee flexion. Passive extension of the seated patient's legs also allows the examiner a quick assessment of hamstring tightness and neural irritation. Stress testing of the knee and ankle is performed to assess ligamentous stability. Any laxity or asymmetry is noted. The sitting position allows for screening of hip flexor, quadricep, hamstring, and foot and ankle strength. A neurovascular screening including testing for motor strength, sensation, reflexes, neural stretch signs (straight leg raising and slump testing), pulse palpation, and measurement of capillary refill is made.

Supine

The supine examination permits a more detailed examination of leg lengths, lower extremity alignment, patellar tracking, and flexibility. The runner performs a bridge maneuver, then the leg lengths are assessed by measuring the distance between the anterior superior iliac spines and the medial malleoli. Discrepancies of even 0.5 to 1.0 cm may be significant in a runner and may require correction.

Assessment of the lower extremity alignment includes determining the degree of femoral and tibial torsion. Femoral torsion is assessed by first palpating the greater trochanter of the leg to be examined. The leg is rotated at the medial and lateral femoral condyles. The other hand positions the greater trochanter in its most lateral position. From this point the relationship between the plane of the femoral condyles to that of the examining table is determined, allowing the examiner to determine the degree of anteversion or retroversion. An anteversion of 8° to 15° is considered normal in the adult.

To assess tibial torsion, the medial and lateral femoral condyles are placed in the frontal plane flat on the table. The examiner then palpates the medial and lateral malleoli. An imaginary axis between the medial and the lateral malleoli is measured against the plane of the examining table. An external tibial rotation of 15° to 25° is considered normal.

The Q angle is formed by the intersection of a line from the anterior superior iliac spine through the midpatella and a secondary imaginary line from the midpatella to the tibial tubercle. A normal Q angle is up to 10° in men and 15° in women. Angles greater than normal may predispose to lateral tracking and patellofemoral pain.

The patella is further assessed by including passive patellar tilt and medial and lateral patellar glide.[11] Passive patellar tilt is assessed by having the examiner place the thumb on the medial edge of the patella and the index finger on the lateral edge. The examiner then tries to elevate the lateral facet from the lateral condyle. The plane of the patella is compared with the axis of the medial and lateral condyles. The tilt is recorded as positive when the lateral edge of the patella rises above the transcondylar axis. Men normally have a tilt of 5° and women 10°. Lesser degrees of tilt may be associated with a tight lateral retinaculum and thus a predisposition to patella tracking problems.

Medial and lateral patellar glides are assessed with the knee resting in 30° of flexion. The patella is longitudinally divided into imaginary quadrants. The patella is then pushed with the thumb medially and laterally. If the medial glide is less than 2 quadrants, a tight lateral restraint is said to be present. A lateral glide of 1 quadrant suggests a competent medial restraint. A lateral glide greater than 3 quadrants suggests an incompetent medial restraint. Patellar apprehension should be noted.

Knee range of motion and stability testing is performed.

The last aspect of the supine biomechanical examination involves testing for adequate lower extremity flexibility. Normal hip flexibility is as follows: flexion is 110° to 120°; extension is 10° to 30°; abduction is 30° to 50°; adduction is 20° to 30°; internal rotation is 30° to 40°; and external rotation is 40° to 60°.[12] The Thomas test assesses hip flexor flexibility.[10] The patient flexes the contralateral hip and knee against the abdomen, with the lumbar spine flat against the table. If the other thigh elevates from the table, a hip flexion contracture is present. Furthermore, in this position the knee should remain flexed to 90°. If the knee passively extends, a tight rectus femoris may be present. Hip internal and external rotation is conveniently assessed with the hip and knee in 90° of flexion.

Hamstring flexibility is also assessed with the hip flexed to 90°. The athlete places both hands in the popliteal space, maintaining this position. The knee is then passively extended as far as possible. In the runner the long axis of the femur and the fibula should have an angle of 180°. Any popliteal angle less than 180° is consistent with hamstring tightness.

Side lying

The side-lying position allows open chain testing of abductor strength (gluteus medius and minimus). The runner should be able to offer resistance during abduction by maintaining the hip in neutral flexion and slight external rotation, thus isolating the gluteals. If the athlete flexes or internally rotates the hip during abduction, a substitution pattern exists.

Flexibility of the iliotibial band (ITB) is measured by the Ober test.[13] The patient is asked to turn on the side facing away from the examiner. The examiner then stabilizes the pelvis and maintains the hip in neutral position. The upper leg is then abducted 30° to 45°, extended at the hip, flexed at the knee, and allowed to passively adduct behind the lower leg. Twenty degrees of cross-adduction is considered normal. Less motion is noted in runners with a tight ITB, tensor fascia lata, or to a lesser degree, tight gluteals.

Prone

The prone position allows a further examination of flexibility, an observation of the soles of the feet, an examination of ankle and foot mobility, and the subtalar neutral examination. To measure quadriceps flexibility the examiner fully flexes the athlete's knee; adequate flexibility is demonstrated if the heel can touch the buttocks. Ankle dorsiflexion is passively assessed with the foot in slight eversion and should be at least 10°.

The examiner then observes the soles of the feet. Excessive wear and abnormal shear forces can be implied by the callus pattern. Dorsiflexion range of motion is noted. Subtalar range of motion is assessed by passively inverting and everting the foot; subtalar mobility is measured. The normal ratio of inversion to eversion is 3:1 with inversion around 30°, and eversion 10°. Midtarsal joint motion is assessed by stabilizing the calcaneus with one hand while inverting and everting the forefoot, comparing for symmetry with the other foot.

The examiner then places the foot in the subtalar neutral position. The examiner remains at the feet of the patient, and with the thumb and index finger, grasps the fourth and fifth metatarsal heads. The thumb and index finger of the other hand are then used to palpate the talar head. When examining the right foot, the examiner's right hand grasps the metatarsal heads, and the left hand appreciates talonavicular congruency. When examining the left foot, the left hand grasps the metatarsal heads, and the right hand finds the subtalar neutral position.

The talus is most easily found by placing the thumb just distal to the medial malleolus at the talonavicular joint, with the middle finger distal to the tibiofibular syndesmosis. The foot is then moved through pronation and supination, with the examiner's thumb appreciating a bulge during pronation, and the index finger feeling a bulge during supination. The neutral position is identified when the bulge is felt equally on both sides. The neutral position, therefore, is that position in which there is talonavicular congruency.

Once subtalar joint neutral is identified, it is possible to establish the relationship of the lower leg to the rear foot and that of the rear foot to the forefoot. To determine the former, the examiner creates imaginary (or water-soluble) lines that bisect the calcaneus and the lower one-third of the lower leg. The relationship is measured with a goniometer. Up to 4° of varus alignment is considered normal.

The relationship of the rear foot to the forefoot is observed. The examiner first ensures that the subtalar joint is in neutral, and the midtarsal joint is pronated by loading the forefoot, which is accomplished by passively dorsiflexing the ankle by exerting a forward pressure on the fourth and fifth metatarsal heads until resistance is felt. The examiner then measures the angle between the bisected calcaneus and an imaginary line is drawn through the heads of the first through fifth metatarsals. The forefoot is neutral if the relationship is perpendicular. If, however, the first metatarsal head lies on a higher plane than the fifth metatarsal head, the forefoot is in a position of varus. If the first metatarsal head is on a lower plane in relationship to the fifth metatarsal head, then there is a forefoot valgus. These measurements can be estimated or determined with a swivel goniometer. The forefoot is normally in a slight varus position of 2° to 3°.

In addition to determining rear foot and forefoot relationships, it is important to assess first ray (first metatarsal) mobility. The range of motion is determined by grasping the heads of the first and the second metatarsals. The first metatarsal is then moved up and down in relationship to the second. The first ray can be rigid, have normal movement, or be hypermobile. A first ray with normal motion can be moved just above and below the second metatarsal. A hypermobile first ray should be aligned with the second through fifth metatarsal heads when assessing the forefoot-rear foot relationship, otherwise the degree of forefoot pronation may be misinterpreted. The prone position also allows for the assessment of hamstring strength by resisting knee flexion and hip extension, and for further examination of the sacroiliac joints and spine with palpation, spring testing, and the femoral stretch test.

Site-Specific Examination

After a thorough biomechanical examination has been performed, the examiner moves on to a site-specific examination. The systematic examination includes the following: inspection, bone palpation, soft tissue palpation, range of motion testing, neurologic examination, specialized testing, and examination of related areas.

Functional Examination

Functional testing assesses the ability of the runner to maintain lower quarter stability. The authors have found 7 tests especially useful: assessment of dynamic pronation or supination, navicular drop, single-legged squat, bilateral squat, the step-down test, star excursion balance test, and swing test. During these maneuvers, the athlete should maintain neutrality in pelvis and leg positioning as well as subtalar neutral positioning at the foot and ankle. Commonly observed defects or compensations include Trendelenburg sign (contralateral dip of the pelvis), a compensated Trendelenburg, forward leaning, and loss of foot and ankle neutrality.

Pronation ↔ supination

Active screening of dynamic pronation/supination should be done in the standing position to assess quantity and quality of subtalar mobility in full weight bearing. Subtalar joint pronation is an integral component in absorbing ground reaction forces during gait. Both the amount and rate of pronation have been associated with overuse running injuries. Instructing the patient to actively roll the arches in and out allows assessment of the following: rear foot inversion and eversion; ability of the midfoot to unlock and contribute to pronation; the ability of the first ray to accept load; the ability of the patient to resupinate, including eversion of the calcaneus; and the ability of the hallux to stabilize with resupination. The rear foot kinematic variables that have most often been associated with overuse running injuries are the amount and rate of foot pronation. Excessive subtalar pronation has been shown to increase stress on tissues within the foot and ankle and has implications up the kinetic chain. An excessive amount of pronation or a change in timing or velocity of pronation has been proposed to require the smaller intrinsic foot muscles and larger extrinsic antipronatory muscles to fire for longer while contracting eccentrically.[14] Limited subtalar eversion can inhibit muscle activation with biomechanical consequences, including increased varus thrust at the knee and prepositioning of the ankle in a more plantar flexed, inverted position at initial contact, a vulnerable position for chronic recurrent sprains. Joint mobilization techniques to restore normal ankle mobility have been shown to improve mechanical faults in those with chronic ankle instability (**Fig. 1**).[15]

Navicular drop
Static navicular drop is described as the change in height of the midpoint of the navicular from subtalar neutral standing to relaxed calcaneal stance. Functional navicular drop is described as the change in navicular height from sitting to standing, not taking subtalar neutral into consideration.[16] A navicular drop of more than 1.5 cm is abnormal and may indicate a heightened need for motion control, through proper footwear, biomechanical orthoses, or pronation-control exercises. An excessive navicular drop has been associated with several running-related injuries including exertional leg pain, medial tibial stress syndrome, compartment syndrome, tibial/fibular or Achilles stress fracture, and tendonopathies (Achilles, peroneal, tibialis anterior and posterior) (**Fig. 2**).[17–21]

Single-leg squat
The single-leg squat is another simple biomechanical screening tool to progressively load the kinetic chain. At the foot, the subtalar joint should be able to stabilize with the initiation of talocrural dorsiflexion. Dynamic knee function is screened as flexion is initiated, assessing the quadriceps ability to eccentrically unlock the knee. The stability of the hip in the frontal and transverse planes and pelvis in the frontal plane is assessed with the single-leg squat.[22,23] In runners with weakness of hip abduction and external rotation, excessive femoral cross-adduction and internal rotation are observed, thus increasing knee valgus moments and dynamic Q angle kinematics associated with athletic injury (**Fig. 3**).

Bilateral squat
The bilateral squat allows further assessment of talocrural and subtalar motion.[24] Full bilateral squat also allows a general screening for intra-articular pathology at the hip and knee. The ability of the talocrural joint to dorsiflex is assessed, observing how

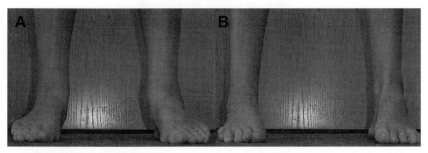

Fig. 1. (*A*) Pronation. (*B*) Supination.

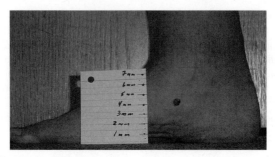

Fig. 2. Navicular drop.

far the athlete can squat prior to early heel rise. Decreased dorsiflexion may result in excessive compensatory pronation and should be corrected if present. Decreased dorsiflexion has also been linked to plantar fasciitis and recurrent ankle sprains in patients with ankle instability (**Fig. 4**).[24–27]

Step-down test

The step-down test seems to be evolving as a simple, defined, objective test with acceptable reliability to assess dynamic hip stability and related neuromuscular

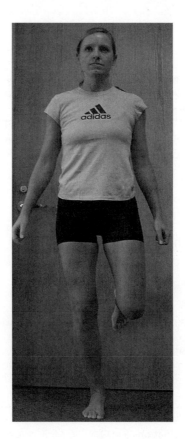

Fig. 3. Single-leg squat.

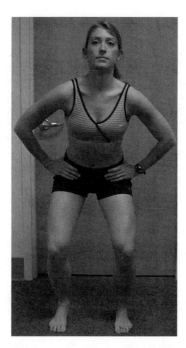

Fig. 4. Bilateral squat.

dysfunction known to be a biomechanical risk factor for common running injuries. A standardized protocol is described as follows: (1) the patient is asked to stand in single-limb support with the hands on the waist, the knee straight, and the foot positioned close to the edge of a 20 cm high step; (2) the contralateral leg is positioned over the floor adjacent to the step and is maintained with the knee in extension; (3) the subject then bends the tested knee until the contralateral leg gently contacts the floor and then reextends the knee to the start position; (4) this maneuver is repeated for 5 repetitions. The examiner faces the subject and scores the test based on 5 criteria:

1. Arm strategy: If subject used an arm strategy in an attempt to recover balance, 1 point is added.
2. Trunk movement: If the trunk leaned to any side, 1 point is added.
3. Pelvis plane: If pelvis rotated or elevated one side compared with the other, 1 point is added.
4. Knee position: If the knee deviates medially and the tibial tuberosity crosses an imaginary vertical line over the second toe, add 1 point, or, if the knee deviates medially and the tibial tuberosity crosses an imaginary vertical line over the medial border of the foot, 2 points are added.
5. Maintain steady unilateral stance: If the subject stepped down on the nontested side, or if the subject's tested limb became unsteady (ie, wavered from side to side on the tested side), add 1 point.

A total score of 0 or 1 is classified as good quality of movement, a total score of 2 or 3 is classified as medium quality, and a total score of 4 or higher is classified as poor quality of movement.[28] The step-down test has been shown to have good correlation with gluteus medius and maximus weakness and knee pain.[29] Souza and Powers[23] reported that individuals with patellofemoral pain syndrome (PFPS) demonstrated 14% less hip abductor strength and 17% less hip external rotator strength with step-down and running, with increased gluteus maximus recruitment. The investigators hypothesized that these individuals with PFPS demonstrated increased activation of gluteals in an attempt to stabilize the hip. Earl and colleagues[30] examined the differences in hip, knee, and ankle kinematics between a bilateral drop-vertical jump and a single-leg step-down. This study found that the unilateral step-down task produces greater motion in the frontal and transverse planes at the ankle and hip, and would be appropriate in evaluating control of the hip during movement. Fredericson and colleagues[31] reported that elite cross-country runners with ITB syndrome demonstrated gluteal weakness and were able to return to prior training level after a specific exercise program targeting on frontal plane strengthening of the hip (**Fig. 5**).

Star Excursion Balance Test

The star excursion balance test (SEBT) is a unilateral balance and reach challenge that incorporates a single-leg squat while reaching with the opposite lower quarter in the sagittal, coronal, and transverse planes. The stance leg requires adequate ankle-dorsiflexion, knee-flexion, and hip-flexion ranges of motion, strength, proprioception, and neuromuscular control to perform these reaching tasks. The patient is instructed to stand on one leg and reach the other foot in front as far as he or she is able to, without touching the ground. The same instruction is given to reach out to 8 total directions 45° from each other in an asterisk pattern. Given the dynamic nature of this assessment and the limited equipment needed, the SEBT holds potential as a cost-effective tool for assessing functional deficits in various common lower extremity conditions in runners.[32]

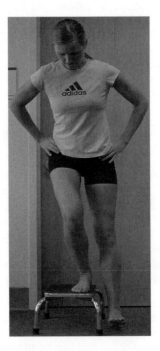

Fig. 5. Step-down test.

Earl and Hertel[33] reported specific muscle activation patterns with specific reach directions. With an anteromedial reach direction vastus medius and lateralis were most activated; with a posterior lateral reach direction, anterior tibialis and biceps femoris were most active; in a posteromedial reach direction, anterior tibialis was most active. More recently, Plisky and colleagues[34] reported that components of the SEBT had good reliability and were predictive measures of lower extremity injury in high school athletes, and suggested that the SEBT can be incorporated into preparticipation physical examinations to help identify neuromuscular patterns in athletes who are at increased risk for injury and design a neuromuscular-based exercise program to improve these deficits.

The SEBT was recently assessed in a chronic ankle instability population. The investigators concluded that the posteromedial, medial, and anteromedial reaches were able to demonstrate significant differences in limbs with chronic ankle instability and those without. The investigators suggest that only a subset of the directions may be needed to assess for chronic ankle instability.[35] The SEBT demonstrated moderate reliability when investigated in 2 previous studies (**Fig. 6**).[33,36]

Swing test

The swing test is a functional dynamic test that is used to assess runners specifically simulating the swing phase of running. The athlete is instructed to stand on a step stool and actively swing the hip through a normal swing phase of running. The swing test is a useful screening tool to assess stance leg stability, swing leg mobility and flexibility, and lumbopelvic stability throughout the swing phase of running mechanics.

Reviews of running lumbopelvic and hip biomechanics have been described.[37–39] Restricted hip flexor or hip joint mobility results in compensation of the lumbar spine

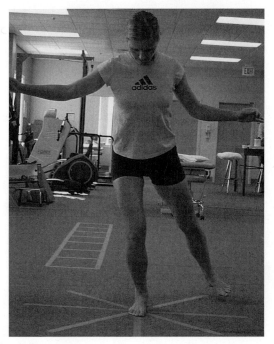

Fig. 6. Star excursion balance test.

(increased lordosis) and pelvis (increased anterior tilt). These compensations may result in poor stability as well as increased eccentric load at the hamstrings, and thus a predisposition to acute injury. Franz and colleagues[38] reported on the relationship between hip extension and anterior pelvic tilt during running and walking. Overall, hip extension and anterior pelvic tilt were greater during running than walking. Anterior pelvic tilt, however, was greater in those with decreased hip extension. The investigators concluded that compensations for the increased stride length during running seem to occur at the pelvis and lumbar spine, rather than at the hip. The study emphasized the clinical relevance regarding the prevention and treatment of hamstring injuries and of injuries to the lumbar spine (**Fig. 7**).

Dynamic evaluation
Subtle abnormalities absent on static examination may become evident with dynamic assessment. Each runner should therefore be examined while both walking and running. Spinal posture, joint motions, and arm and leg swing are assessed. Balance is noted at the shoulder, pelvis, hips, knees, feet, and ankles, recognizing the relationship throughout the kinetic chain. Any asymmetries are recorded and assessed for contributing factors. Antalgia is always significant.

Video gait analysis is generally reserved for recalcitrant cases and can be useful in identifying subtle imbalances in alignment, flexibility, strength, and mobility. Athletes should be familiar and comfortable with treadmill running. Video analysis should include whole body assessment in multiple planes to examine the entire kinetic chain in addition to foot and ankle mechanics.

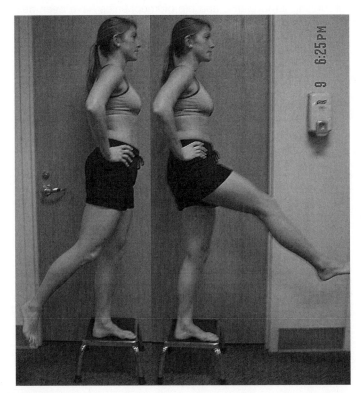

Fig. 7. Swing test.

Shoe evaluation

The runner is encouraged to bring in for examination all previously used running shoes. The shoes should be examined for specific wear patterns. Most runners heel strike on the lateral aspect of the heel, so wear in the posterolateral heel is not uncommon. Excessive lateral heel wear, however, can lead to excessive varus load with subsequent lateral knee pain. Determinations about the runner's degree of pronation and supination are best made by examining the forefoot.

Excessive pronation causes excessive wear along the medial forefoot. Wear in the midsection of the forefoot indicates a probable normal toe-off. Wear on the lateral side is indicative of a runner with supinated gait. Excessive pronation is additionally accomplished by a medially tilted heel counter, whereas a supinated gait causes the heel counter to tilt laterally.

The shoes are additionally assessed for the type of last and construction. Unique combinations of last and construction offer varying degrees of motion control and shock absorbency. Quality control is also inspected by examining areas of the shoe that require gluing or stitching.

SUMMARY

The injured runner is one of the most challenging athletes the sports medicine physician will encounter. A comprehensive history and biomechanical examination assists the practitioner in diagnosing and managing running injuries successfully. The extra time and effort that is afforded to the initial evaluation provides the runner the best opportunity to return to running and remain injury free.

REFERENCES

1. Wilder RP, O'Connor F. Evaluation of the injured runner. In: O'Connor F, Wilder R, editors. The textbook of running medicine. New York: McGraw-Hill; 2001. p. 45–58.
2. Wilder R, O'Connor F, Barrish W. Biomechanical evaluation of the injured runner. Biomechanics 2001;8:24–41.
3. O'Connor F, Wilder R. Evaluation of the injured runner. J Back Musculoskelet Rehabil 1995;5:281.
4. O'Connor FG, Sobel JR, Nirschl RP. Five-step treatment for overuse injuries. Phys Sportsmed 1992;20:128–42.
5. Leadbetter WB. Cell-matrix response in tendon injury. Clin Sports Med 1992;11: 533–78.
6. Macintyre JG, Lloyd-Smith DR. Overuse running injuries. In: Renstrom PA, editor. Sports injury—basic principles of prevention and care. Boston: Blackwell Scientific Publications; 1993. p. 139–60.
7. Brody DM. Evaluation of the injured runner. Tech Orthop 1990;5:15–22.
8. When the feet hit the ground everything changes. Toledo (OH): American Physical Rehabilitation Network; 1986. Basic course.
9. Drez D. Examination of the lower extremity in runners. In: D'Ambrosia RD, Drez D, editors. Prevention and treatment of running injuries. Thorofare (NJ): Slack Incorporated; 1989. p. 36–41.
10. Magee DJ. Orthopedic physical assessment. Philadelphia: WB Saunders Company; 1992. p. 319–20.
11. Paulos LE, Kolowich PA. Patellar instability and pain. In: Reider B, editor. Sports medicine: the school age athlete. Philadelphia: WB Saunders Company; 1991. p. 332–53.

12. Hoppenfeld S. Physical examination of the spine and extremities. East Norwalk (CT): Appleton-Century-Crofts; 1976.

13. Ober FB. The role of the iliotibial and fascia lata as a factor in the causation of low-back disabilities and sciatica. J Bone Joint Surg 1936;18:105.

14. Tweed JL, Campbell JA, Avil SJ. Biomechanical risk factors in the development of medial tibial stress syndrome in distance runners. J Am Podiatr Med Assoc 2008; 98(6):436–44.

15. Green T, Refshauge K, Crosbie J, et al. A randomized controlled trial of a passive accessory joint mobilization on acute ankle inversion sprains. Phys Ther 2001;81: 984–94.

16. Hesar NG, Ginkel AV, Cools A, et al. A prospective study on gait-related intrinsic risk factors for lower leg overuse injuries. Br J Sports Med 2009;43:1–11.

17. Reinking MF. Exercise-related leg pain in female collegiate athletes: the influence of intrinsic and extrinsic factors. Am J Sports Med 2006;34:1500–7.

18. Kaufman KR, Brodine SK, Shaffer RA, et al. The effect of foot structure and range of motion on musculoskeletal overuse injuries. Am J Sports Med 1999; 27:585.

19. Molloy JM, Douglas CS, Teyhen DS, et al. Effect of running shoe type on the distribution and magnitude of plantar pressures in individuals with low- or high-arched feet. J Am Podiatr Med Assoc 2009;99(4):330–8.

20. Bennett JE, Reinking MF, Pluemer B, et al. Factors contributing to the development of medial tibial stress syndrome in high school runners. J Orthop Sports Phys Ther 2001;31(9):504–10.

21. Plisky MS, Rauh MJ, Heiderscheit B, et al. Medial tibial stress syndrome in high school cross-country runners: incidence and risk factors. J Orthop Sports Phys Ther 2007;37(2):40–7.

22. Willson JD, Ireland ML, Davis I. Core strength and lower extremity alignment during single leg squats. Med Sci Sports Exerc 2006;38(5):945–52.

23. Souza RB, Powers CM. Differences in hip kinematics, muscle strength, and muscle activation between subjects with and without patellofemoral pain. J Orthop Sports Phys Ther 2009;39(1):12–9.

24. Cornwall MW, McPoil TG. Effect of ankle dorsiflexion range of motion on rear foot motion during walking. J Am Podiatr Med Assoc 1999;89:272–7.

25. Warren B, Jones CJ. Predicting plantar fasciitis in runners. Med Sci Sports Exerc 1987;19:71–3.

26. Kwong PK, Kay D, Voner RT, et al. Plantar fasciitis: mechanics and pathomechanics of treatment. Clin Sports Med 1988;7:119–26.

27. Drewes LK, McKeon PO, Casey Kerrigan D, et al. Dorsiflexion deficit during jogging with chronic ankle instability. J Sci Med Sport 2009;12:685–7.

28. Piva SR, Fitzgerald K, Irrgang JJ, et al. Reliability of measures of impairments associated with patellofemoral pain syndrome. BMC Musculoskelet Disord 2006;7:33.

29. Hollman JH, Ginos BE, Kozuchowski J, et al. Relationships between knee valgus, hip-muscle strength, and hip-muscle recruitment during a single-limb step-down. J Sport Rehabil 2009;18(1):104–17.

30. Earl JE, Monteiro SK, Snyder KR. Differences in lower extremity kinematics between a bilateral drop-vertical jump and a single-leg step-down. J Orthop Sports Phys Ther 2007;37(5):245–52.

31. Fredericson M, Cookingham CL, Chaudhari AM, et al. Hip abductor weakness in distance runners with iliotibial band syndrome. Clin J Sport Med 2000;10(3): 169–75.

32. Olmstead LC, Carcia CR, Hertel J, et al. Efficacy of the star excursion balance tests in detecting reach deficits in subjects with chronic ankle instability. J Athl Train 2002;37(4):501–6.
33. Earl JE, Hertel J. Lower-extremity muscle activation during the star excursion balance tests. J Sport Rehabil 2001;10:93–104.
34. Plisky PJ, Rauh MJ, Kaminski TW, et al. Star excursion balance test as a predictor of lower extremity injury in high school basketball players. J Orthop Sports Phys Ther 2006;36(12):911–9.
35. Hertel J, Braham RA, Hale SA, et al. Simplifying the star excursion balance test: analyses of subjects with and without chronic ankle instability. J Orthop Sports Phys Ther 2006;36(3):131–7.
36. Hertel J, Miller SJ, Denegar CR. Intratester and intertester reliability during the Star Excursion Balance Tests. J Sport Rehabil 2000;9:104–16.
37. Schache AG, Bennell KL, Blanch PD, et al. The coordinated movement of the lumbo-pelvic-hip complex during running: a literature review. Gait Posture 1999;10(1):30–47.
38. Franz JR, Paylo KW, Dicharry J, et al. Changes in the coordination of hip and pelvis kinematics with mode of locomotion. Gait Posture 2009;29(3):494–8.
39. Chumanov ES, Heiderscheit BC, Thelen DG. The effect of speed and influence of individual muscles on hamstring mechanics during the swing phase of sprinting. J Biomech 2007;40(16):3555–62.

Kinematics and Kinetics of Gait: From Lab to Clinic

Jay Dicharry, MPT

KEYWORDS

• Gait • Kinematics • Kinetics • Running

The ultimate goal of gait analysis is to understand the relationship between an individual's functional capabilities and limitations and gait pattern, with the purpose of enhancing performance while preventing injury.[1] The physiologic aspects of training the running athlete are well-known. The biomechanical variables associated with training are less understood by clinicians. This article reviews the components of gait and helps clinicians apply these concepts to clinical analysis.

Human locomotion involves moving a center of mass (COM) across a given distance. Gait can be monitored subjectively in the clinic, or can be quantified objectively in a modern three-dimensional (3D) gait laboratory setting. The selected method must be able to assess the desired parameters. The relatively young science of biomechanical gait analysis, combined with the inherent variability of individual runners, makes the comprehensive study of running gait challenging.[2,3] A clinical gait evaluation, however, used in conjunction with a thorough history, physical examination, and functional screen is a powerful tool for shedding light on the dysfunction causing an individual's symptoms.

THE GAIT CYCLE

The gait cycle describes the time and space parameters that occur in the distinctly different activities of walking and running.[4] The lower body limbs experience both stance and swing periods, but the timing and contact patterns of these stance and swing phases differentiate the two tasks of walking and running. Stance phase begins at contact with the ground. Swing phase initiates as that limb moves into toe-off. The walking gait cycle has a period of double support (both feet in contact with the ground at the same time) and a period of single-leg support. An individual is able to walk at varied speeds while still maintaining these essential characteristics, and as evidenced by the rapid pace of elite race-walkers. Gait is described as running when the gait cycle exhibits single-leg support and double-leg float (flight) periods. Therefore,

The Center for Endurance Sport, Department of Physical Medicine and Rehabilitation, The University of Virginia, 545 Ray C. Hunt Drive, Suite 240, Charlottesville, VA 22903, USA
E-mail address: jd4da@virginia.edu

Clin Sports Med 29 (2010) 347–364
doi:10.1016/j.csm.2010.03.013
0278-5919/10/$ – see front matter © 2010 Elsevier Inc. All rights reserved.

walkers always have at least one limb in contact with the ground, and runners either have one limb or no limbs in contact with the ground at respective periods of gait.

Gait cycles can be categorized. The walking gait is subdivided into eight distinct phases: initial contact, loading response, midstance, terminal stance, preswing, initial swing, midswing, and terminal swing (**Fig. 1**). Although these distinct periods offer a method to categorize gait, they can be combined to reflect the three functional components for each limb: (1) weight acceptance (initial contact, loading response), (2) single limb support (midstance, terminal swing, preswing), and (3) limb advancement (initial swing, midswing, terminal swing). The first two functional components occur during the stance phases with the third occurring during swing. Running gait cycles are broken down into the following phases: stance phase absorption, stance phase generation, swing phase generation, swing phase reversal, and swing phase absorption. The stance phase is typically emphasized in most clinical running observation and can be broken down into (1) initial contact to foot flat, (2) foot flat to heel-off, and (3) heel-off to toe-off.

Definition of temporal–spatial gait parameters allows objective reports of both walking and running; they define where, when, how long, and how rapidly the individual is in contact with the ground. These parameters include stride time, step time, stride length, step length, gait velocity, and cadence. Stride time is the time from initial contact of one foot to initial contact of the same foot. Step time refers to the period of initial contact of one foot to initial contact of the opposite foot. Stride length is the distance covered between initial contact of one foot to initial contact of the same foot, whereas step length reflects the distance form initial contact of one limb to the initial contact of the opposite limb. Gait velocity is stride length divided by stride time, usually expressed as meters per second or miles per hour. Cadence refers to the number of steps taken in a unit of time, usually expressed as steps per

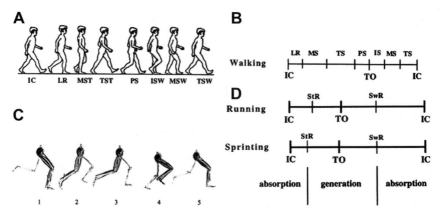

Fig. 1. The gait cycle. (*A*) Walking figure. IC, initial contact; ISW, initial swing; LR, loading response; MST, midstance; MSW, midswing; PS, preswing; TST, terminal stance; TSW, terminal swing. (*B*) Walking gait cycle. IC, initial contact; LR, loading response; IS, initial swing; MS (first instance), midstance; MS (second instance), midswing; PS, preswing; TO, toe off; TS (first instance), terminal stance; TS (second instance), terminal swing. (*C*). Running figure. 1. Stance phase absorption. 2. Stance phase generation. 3. Swing phase generation. 4. Swing phase reversal. 5. Swing phase absorption. (*D*) Running gait cycle for running and sprinting. Absorption, from SwR through IC to StR; generation, from StR through TO to SwR. IC, initial contact; StR, stance phase reversal; SwR, swing phase reversal; TO, toe off. (*From* Novacheck TF. The biomechanics of running. Gait Posture 1998;7:77–95; with permission.)

minute. These characteristics can be monitored with pressure mats, force platforms, and 3D motion analysis camera systems. Foot switches (on/off devices to collect foot contact timing) allow temporal data to be collected but ignore spatial data.

During the walking gait cycle, approximately 60% of time is spent in stance phase and 40% in swing. Under average walking speeds, each double-limb support comprises 10% of the gait cycle (total, 20%), whereas single-limb stance accounts for the remaining 80% of stance phase. During slower walking speeds the double-limb support phase increases, whereas faster walking speeds reflect shorter double-limb support periods (**Fig. 2**).[3,5] Running reverses the support characteristics found in walking: less than 40% of the gait cycle is spent in stance and greater than 60% is spent in swing. As running speed increases, the time spent in stance decreases and that spent in swing increases. To increase speed, an initial increase occurs in step length, followed by increased cadence. Increased stride length is associated with an increase in velocity and is limited by leg length and the athlete's ability to generate sufficient force to move the COM forward. Although cadence is trainable, its direct impact on ground contact time, and thus ground reaction forces (GRFs) acting on the runner, reflect that a preferred cadence might be a protective effect to stem both impact forces and loading rates.[6] Typical values for cadence vary from the low 70s to the mid-90s for all runners, including distance runners and sprinters. **Fig. 2** illustrates the relationship of stance time to swing time throughout various speeds.[3]

KINEMATICS OF GAIT

The study of kinematics involves the use of 3D motion analysis systems that digitally reconstruct the individual's body as a multisegment system. After infrared markers are placed at specific anatomic landmarks, their position is triangulated by cameras to calibrate the individual into the system. Construction of the coordinates and orientation of the rigid body segments allow calculation of joint angles of the proximal and distal segment, joint angular velocity, and joint acceleration. Measurements are collected for each joint in all three cardinal planes of motion. Movement of the COM of each body segment impacts the overall COM of the individual, which is critical for balance and energy expenditure.[1] During walking, the COM trajectory is at the highest point in stance, when speed is minimum. During running, the COM reaches

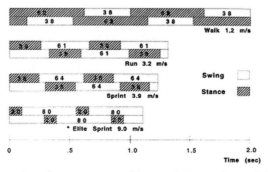

Fig. 2. Variation in gait cycle parameters with speed. For each condition, the bar graph begins at initial contact on the left and represents two complete gait cycles or strides. Note that as speed increases, time spent in swing (*clear*) increases, stance time (*shaded*) decreases, double float increases, and cycle time shortens. (*From* Novacheck TF. The biomechanics of running. Gait Posture 1998;7:77–95; with permission.)

the highest point in the flight phase, when velocity is maximum.[5] Although skin artifact is inherent in this data collection process, modern 3D motion analysis systems currently represent the most noninvasive tool for reliable kinematic data collection.[2,7–11]

Running-joint kinematic patterns differ somewhat from those of walking. Differences are more pronounced in the sagittal plane and somewhat muted in the coronal and transverse planes. However, absolute peak values are not always the primary focus of an analysis, because they are also greatly influenced by the athlete's training level and speed. The timing of the extremes of mobility (and force data presented in the following section) is a more important descriptor because it better exemplifies individual characteristics.[3] Although 3D gait analysis produces graphs for each plane of motion of each specific joint (**Fig. 3**), all body segments are coupled in a closed kinetic chain during stance and an open kinetic chain in swing.

Sagittal Plane Kinematics

As the body transitions from walking to running to sprinting, the COM is lowered and the body tilt in space shifted forward. The combined effect is to maximize the propulsion phase. Although Novacheck reported that pelvic orientation stays remarkably similar to maintain economy,[3] recent studies have shown changes in pelvic orientation with running.

Using healthy adult subjects, Franz and colleagues[12] recently showed that despite an increased stride length in running, hip range of motion is unchanged from walking to running. Instead, the compensations in sagittal plane involved an increase in anterior pelvic tilt and thigh angle (thigh-in-space angle). Furthermore, they observed a greater anterior pelvic tilt in subjects who displayed reduced utilized peak hip extension. Thus, this limitation of hip flexor mobility shifts pelvic orientation and may place the lumbar spine in a compromised position for core muscle activation and have implications for low-back pain.[13] Both Chumanov and colleagues[14] and Thelen and colleagues[15] report that this altered pelvic orientation and relationship between the hip flexors and extensors may also place additional strain on the hamstrings. Preservation of pelvic alignment during running is a key variable to consider in these injury populations.

In walking, the hip shows peak extension just before toe-off and peak flexion in mid- to terminal swing. In running, the peak range of extension is similar to that of walking; however, peak extension occurs at toe-off. Increased peak hip flexion is seen during running to advance the limb in swing. Overall hip flexion/extension and abduction/adduction mobility are increased in running (approximately 60° and 15°, respectively) compared with walking (approximately 40° and 10°, respectively).

Unlike in walking, in running the hip must extend in the later part of swing so as to place the foot in the correct orientation under the body. If this did not occur, foot contact would be too far ahead of the COM and shift the GRFs posterior, thus causing deceleration. Correct hip position at contact can be best visualized as riding on a skateboard or scooter. Planting the stance leg close to the COM at contact tends to preserve the GRF close to the COM and minimize the deceleration component. Placing the foot excessively anterior will cause an abrupt braking force. This characteristic is accentuated in sprinters in that the hip in a more extended position at contact will continue to produce net acceleration with the COM ahead of the contact limb.

The knee exhibits similar patterns in walking and running, flexing once to absorb in stance and once to clear the limb in swing. Although the patterns are the same, the amount of knee flexion in swing increases greatly from approximately 60° in walking to upwards of 90° in running. Some sprinters achieve 105° to 130° of knee flexion in

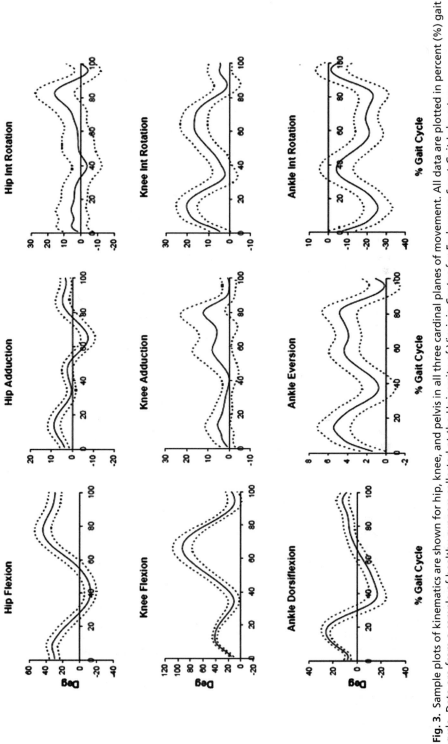

Fig. 3. Sample plots of kinematics are shown for hip, knee, and pelvis in all three cardinal planes of movement. All data are plotted in percent (%) gait cycle. Data are from a sample of healthy runners collected at the University of Virginia Center for Endurance Sport Gait Laboratory.

swing. In stance, the running knee is flexed approximately 25° at contact and continues flexing to 45° peak in midstance. Less peak flexion in stance occurs in sprinters because of the lower ground contact time.

In walking, the tibia is positioned so that the contact is made at the heel with the ankle in plantar flexion. The position of the tibia is more vertical in running, requiring more dorsiflexion of the ankle to achieve contact. Moving past initial contact, the walking ankle initially plantar flexes to achieve foot flat, whereas the running ankle moves into dorsiflexion as the limb is loaded. Because of shorter contact times, sprinters tend to run more on the forefoot, and thus have less peak dorsiflexion at the ankle in midstance. Moving into propulsion, sprinters have increased plantar flexion at toe-off and decreased need for dorsiflexion to clear the limb in swing because of increased mobility of the knee.

To summarize, net ankle mobility is higher in running (50°) than walking (30°). The timing of peak ankle values occur earlier in the stance phase as running speed increases.

Full dorsiflexion of the metatarsal joints (normally 85°) is not needed for walking or running; however, a limitation (<30° metatarsophalangeal [MTP] at the first ray) can cause significant changes. A significant amount of leverage, and thus stability, is provided from the first ray and its musculotendinous structures from late stance through toe-off. An individual with restricted MTP extension cannot rollover through the metatarsal heads at toe-off, causing the foot to supinate early and thus shifting the base of support laterally on the foot away from the stable first ray. This process introduces a "heel whip" into the gait cycle that forces rotational motion into the entire kinetic chain.

A clinical examination performed with the ankle in a relaxed plantar flexed position can reveal arthrokinematic restriction in mobility of the MTP joints. However, all of the lower leg tissues are continuous in nature. Assessing MTP mobility with the ankle in slight dorsiflexion better replicates the position of the ankle at toe-off and offers the unique ability to examine the combined effects of the calf musculature, Achilles, and plantar fascia together. A limitation in one or all of these structures can limit mobility of the MTP even when the joint itself might move freely. Identification and treatment of the soft tissue structure at fault allows unimpeded progression of the runner through the forefoot.

Coronal and Transverse Plane Kinematics

Motion in the mediolateral direction during walking and running is more subtle than in the sagittal plane. Nonsagittal plane mobility in gait acts to moderate stability, force attenuation, and economy in gait. Motions of pronation and supination are visualized not as isolated events occurring only in the foot, but as an interconnected multiseg-ment system that functions together. An alteration in one specific location can impact the joints both above or below that segment. **Table 1** summarizes the coupled motions occurring in the lower quarter during the pronation and supination phases.

The hip adducts relative to the pelvis during the stance phase and is abducted relative to the pelvis during the swing phase.[3] Thus, if the runner is on the right foot during midstance, the right hip will be adducted, the contralateral side of the pelvis will be lower, and the lumbar spine will be slightly side bent to the right side. This coupled motion between the hip, pelvis and lumbar spine acts to minimize motion to the trunk and head for balance and equilibrium.

Although some mobility here is beneficial, too much or too little may cause additional problems. Step width may influence this motion, because a crossover or adducted gait may induce excessive pelvic drop on the contralateral side. Weak hip

Table 1
The effects of pronation and supination on the kinetic chain

	Pronation			Supination		
	Sagittal	Frontal	Transverse	Sagittal	Frontal	Transverse
Lumbosacral	Extension	Lat Flexion Same Side	Protraction	Extension	Lat Flexion Opp Side	Retraction
Pelvis	Anterior rotation	Translation and elevation, same side	Forward rot same side	Anterior rotation	Translation opp side; depression same side	Rear rot same side
Hip	Flexion	Adduction	Internal rotation	Extension	Abduction	External rotation
Knee	Flexion	Abduction	Internal rotation	Extension	Adduction	External rotation
Ankle	PF-DF		Internal rotation	DF-PF		External rotation
STJ	PF	Eversion	Adduction	DF	Inversion	Abduction
MTJ	DF	Inversion	Abduction	PF	Eversion	Adduction

Abbreviations: DF, dorsiflexion; Lat, lateral; MTJ, midtalar joint; Opp, opposite; PF, plantarflexion; rot, rotation; STJ, subtalar joint.
Data from Dugan SA, Bhat KP. Biomechanics and analysis of running gait. Phys Med Rehabil Clin N Am 2005;16(3):603–21; with permission.

abductors can cause increased hip adduction and pelvic drop (Trendelenberg). Weak hip stability can also lead to a compensatory lateral trunk shift to move COM laterally and limit pelvic drop. Altered hip stability recruitment patterns decrease running economy and have been shown to be associated with injury, including patellofemoral dysfunction.[16,17] Too little motion, with little to no adduction between the hip and pelvis, can also be problematic. Although commonly seen when sprinting all out, this should not be a goal of typical gait. Additionally, too little motion may require additional stabilization at the knee (high metabolic cost) or contribute to inadequate shock transmission. For example, using a wide stance width with little coronal plane mobility at the hip and pelvis can lead to decreased shock absorption. This positioning could create a situation where additional forces could be transferred to the pelvis. Problem-solving through this unique combination of gait attributes can show the biomechanical flaws placing additional stress at the pelvis and thus contributing to an injury such as osteitis pubis or sacral stress fractures. If the cause of this gait abnormality is not corrected in the run technique, the abnormal loading pattern will persist and conditions will become repeat or chronic.

Foot and ankle mechanics are a critical aspect of the evaluation. The foot and ankle function as a mobile lever. Their ability to move into an open packed position (full pronation) to absorb and dissipate shock is critical to achieve contact and avoid excessive shock transmission up the kinematic chain. Likewise, the foot must be able to resupinate at the correct time in push-off to maximize force transfer.

In a clinical setting, barefoot gait evaluation can yield a plethora of information about the foot, but clinicians must be aware of the complex foot mechanics.[18] In running, it is typically taught that the foot moves from a supinated position at contact (in 6°–8° calcaneal inversion) into 6° to 8° eversion at midstance, and then immediately begins to supinate into a more rigid state.[1] This premise was based largely on using rearfoot mobility to define the pronatory status of the foot. McPoil and Cornwall[19] accordingly note that rearfoot pronation peaks at 37.9% of stance phase of walking. Recent work has shown that using the rearfoot to define the pronatory status of the foot may be less specific than using a dynamic foot measurement with motion analysis. Peak composite foot deformation does not occur until approximately 78% of stance in walking and until 52% to 54% in running.[20] Maximal deformation of the foot in the gait cycle occurs at maximal GRF application.

KINETICS OF GAIT

Although kinematics can be visually evaluated in the laboratory and clinic, they do not show why individuals move the way they do. Kinetics reflect the cause of movement, and therefore the forces, power, and energy that affect the manner in which an individual moves.[21] GRFs measured with force plates imbedded in the ground or treadmill refer to the forces that act on the body throughout the stance phase.[22] Analysis of the GRFs acting on the COM is typically broken down into vertical, mediolateral, and anteroposterior force plots (**Fig. 4**). The origin of force on the foot is termed *center of pressure* (COP). Processing the COP, GRFs, and joint kinematics together allows calculation of joint kinetics (joint moments). More specifically, joint kinetics show how the external GRFs, inertia, and gravity interact with the internal recruitment of muscles, tendons, ligaments, and bony structures that stabilize the joint. Joint power indicates the velocity of the joint moment, or the rate of the work exhibited by the muscles. Although monitoring kinetics is not possible outside a laboratory setting, understanding these attributes helps clinicians appreciate why runners move the way they do at various points in the gait cycle.

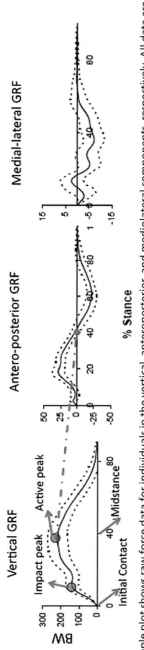

Fig. 4. Sample plot shows raw force data for individuals in the vertical, anteroposterior, and mediolateral components, respectively. All data are plotted in percent stance, with percent body weight (BW) as the unit of measure. For the vertical ground reaction force (GRF), the first peak represents the collision of shoe and lower leg with the ground. The magnitude of the impact varies greatly with contact style, cadence, and slope of the running surface. The more prominent second represents active peak; this is the point in the gait cycle where external forces acting on the body are at their peak, thus triggering maximum internal force generation of the musculotendinous structures to balance this response. Note that the active peak on the vertical GRF always corresponds to the "0" point on the anteroposterior GRF as long as speed is at steady state. Data are from a sample of healthy runners collected at the University of Virginia Center for Endurance Sport Gait Laboratory.

The vertical GRF has two distinct peaks for walking gait and one distinct peak for running. With an average comfortable walking speed, the GRF spikes at initial contact to form a small impact peak, and then increases through the absorption phase peak to approximately 100% to 110% body weight, dips to approximately 80% COM in double support, and finally increases back to approximately 100% to 110% in the force generation phase. Thus, in walking, the typical peak vertical forces are similar to those experienced in a single-leg stance. During running, vertical GRF spikes sharply at contact to produce an impact peak, may slightly decrease (depending on contact style), and then continues to an active peak of 2.2 to 2.6 times the body weight in a typical distance runner.

The impact peak is formed through collision of the shoe, foot, and lower leg mass with the ground. The active peak is influenced by the mass of the runner, landing velocity, and leg stiffness.[23] The presence of an impact peak, or its prominence, can be moderated by alteration in contact style. Runners with a more pronounced heel contact exhibit larger impact peaks, whereas sprinters or toe runners may have no discernable impact peak. Cadence also has an effect, with increased turnover exhibiting muted or even absent impact peaks, and decreased turnover accentuating impact peaks.[24] Cadence change has been shown to be a clinically significant component of a plan to decrease the incidence of bone-strain–related injury.[25] Gottschall and Kram[23] reported that impact force peaks were dramatically larger for downhill running and smaller for uphill running.

Do increased impact forces lead to injury or impact performance? Hreljac[26,27] is widely cited as identifying impact peak force as the variable that distinguished injured from uninjured runners. However, this concept has been sharply contested by Nigg,[28] who states that impact forces help in pre-tension, or tuning the muscle contraction of the leg before impact. Furthermore, some level of impact force is necessary for the integrity of bone and cartilage.[29] Nigg[28] does speculate, however, that excessive running without sufficient recovery may adversely affect the remodeling rate of bone. Impact peak forces are comparatively small and experienced for a short time during each gait cycle (<8% of each stance phase). Joint contact forces during the impact peak are three to five times smaller than they are during the active force peak, and are therefore within the normal operating ranges for joint function and unlikely to contribute to the development of running injury.[30]

As depicted by the vertical GRF graphs (see **Fig. 4**), peak forces on the body are sustained during midstance, not initial contact. The active force peak of the vertical GRF reflects the number of motor units required to hold the body at a given point and occurs at the lowest point of the COM in the stance phase.[24,31–33] Decreased active peak for the same speed means a decrease in motor unit activation and metabolic demand to hold speed.[32] The active peak of the GRF can be modified through mass, velocity of the runner, and contact time.[32,33] Unlike the impact peak, the active peak is not altered with incline or decline as long as steady state velocity is maintained.[23]

Midstance is the time in the gait cycle when GRFs are highest on the body, with peak internal joint moments generating peak mechanical strain on tissues. The ability of the runner to stabilize these forces is essential to tissue health. Dynamic screening tests performed in single-leg stance offer a functional and running specific midstance posture from which to evaluate stability. From a rehabilitation standpoint, challenging a runner's multiplane stability in single-leg stance replicates the position and phase in gait at which it is most critical.

In addition to vertical GRF, the anteroposterior (or parallel forces) and mediolateral GRFs are analyzed to describe the sagittal and frontal plane forces, respectively.

Assuming the runner is at steady state, the active peak corresponds to the "0" point on the x axis. Any negative value will then decelerate the COM, with positive values accelerating the COM. At steady state velocity, the time-integrated brake force equals the propulsive force so that minimum mechanical efficiency is lost. Anteroposterior GRF can be altered through contact style, cadence, or incline so that braking peak increases for running downhill and decreases for running uphill. Likewise, propulsion force increases in uphill running and decreases in downhill running.[23] Excessively elevated parallel braking forces can indicate that the individual's COM is well behind the foot at contact. This tendency can be remedied by encouraging a more neutral postural alignment and foot strike closer to the COM.

Mediolateral GRF allows quantification of the path of the COM in the frontal plane. Excessive deviation from medial to lateral (or lateral to medial) imparts excess coronal plane forces that the runner is required to stabilize. Increased deviation in this plane is often seen when the runner lacks adequate hip and core stability. This increased instability of COM combined with poor neuromuscular control can lead to a "downward spiral" in the stance. Efforts should target identification of the biomechanical fault and be combined with gait drills to minimize the peak deviation of COM in relation to the stance foot.

Joint Kinetics

Quantitatively, motion laboratories use inverse dynamics to combine kinematics and external GRF to produce joint moments and powers. The ability to conceptualize the joint moment at each specific gait phase helps in applying a clinical and dynamic evaluation to a gait analysis. The GRF has a given magnitude for a given gait phase. Additionally, this vector has a point of origin or COP and direction in relation to each joint. The location of this vector dictates what the external GRF is doing to the joint, and what the runner is doing to counter this action. For example, during midstance, the ankle joint is in dorsiflexion and the GRF is anterior to the ankle joint line (**Fig. 5**). The GRF is imposing an external torque trying to dorsiflex the ankle, while the runner activates the plantar flexors to generate an equal and opposite internal joint torque to maintain position of the ankle at that particular point in time. At any instance in stance, three factors influence the joint kinetics: (1) the magnitude of the GRF, (2) the 3D GRF location in relation to the joint, and (3) the origin of the COP (influenced by foot contact style or compensatory foot function). **Fig. 6** shows sample graphs of running joint kinetics in healthy young adults.

The origin of COP is affected by contact style. Because rear-foot runners land on the posterolateral border of the foot, the origin of COP initiates on the lateral aspect of the foot and travels distal for two thirds of the stance phase before traveling medial across the metatarsal heads and finally through the first and second rays.[34] Midfoot strikers' COP originates on the lateral midfoot, with an initial path posterior toward the base of the foot as the rearfoot approximates the ground. After maximum foot contact, the COP moves rapidly toward the medial forefoot. Forefoot strikers share this same general pattern, except that the initial COP origin is even more distal on the foot.[35]

These described paths are typical values, but compensations can occur because of foot mechanics. An individual who has poor forefoot stability may have an excessive lateral to medial COP shift as he moves into propulsion phase, whereas the COP of an individual with hallux rigidus will track more lateral and exit through the lateral forefoot.

Rise and fall of the COM occurs during walking and running; however, this action yields different results in each task. In walking, kinetic and potential energy are out of phase so that COM moves from its highest point in single-leg stance to its lowest point in double-leg stance. This pendulum-like oscillation of the COM is maintained

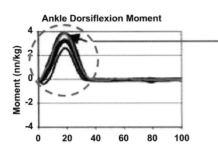
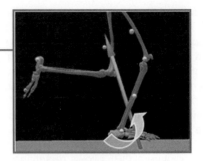

The GRF induces an <u>external</u> <u>dorsiflexion</u> <u>moment</u> at the ankle

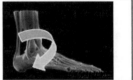

<u>Internal plantarflexion</u> <u>moment</u> counters this external moment

Fig. 5. External and internal factors that effect joint kinetics at the ankle.

by the interchange of potential and kinetic energy and, combined with a given amount of muscle work, propels the body. During running, the body acts like a pogo stick in that potential and kinetic energy are in phase. Potential and kinetic energy are highest in the flight phase. Potential energy is lost as the body falls down to the ground. Kinetic energy is lost as the foot achieves ground contact, but is stored in the musculotendinous structures as elastic energy. After midstance, the tendon springs release approximately 95% of their stored energy in combination with tensioning from the muscles to generate the COM upward and thus raise potential and kinetic energy back to their high point. This storage and rebound of the tendon units is an important component of running gait, because they supply most of the work performed.[3,36]

Although the muscles act as tensioners to the tendons, they do not exhibit much of a change in length. Rather, uniarticular muscles stabilize joints, whereas biarticular muscles transfer energy to adjacent joints.[37,38] The gluteus medius is an example of a uniarticular muscle. The gluteus medius exhibits tension during the stance phase to hold the pelvis stable, although it does not undergo a significant change in muscle length. When looking at a biarticular example, the energy from one segment is transferred through the "energy strap" so that the energy of the femur extending over the tibia can be transferred through the hamstrings to extend the hip in relation to the pelvis.[3]

During walking, a great deal of mechanical work is dissipated at each contact point because of collision of the foot with the ground.[39,40] The contralateral trailing limb restores this energy and the velocity of COM, but the difference must be made up from active muscle work (significant muscle change in length) that is not seen in running. In running, a major energy expense seems to be due to body weight support. The overly flexed position of the knee (compared with walking) increases the joint moment and the knee extensor demand.[41,42] During running, the stiffness of the stance leg spring may be altered as much as twofold to adapt either to cadence changes outside the individual's preferred frequency, or to the surface so that stability

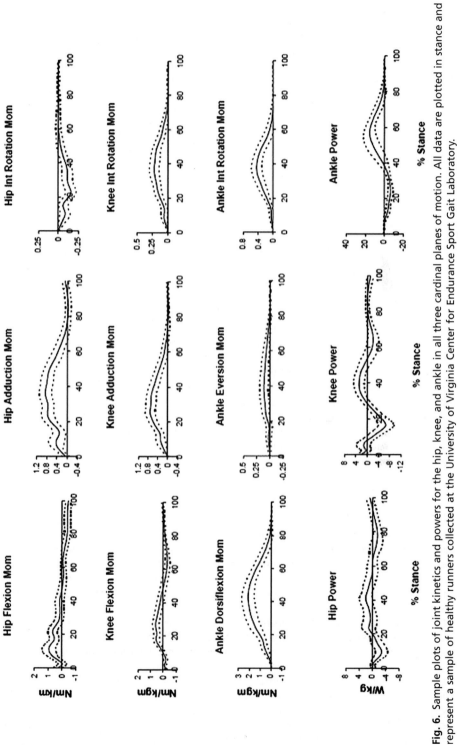

Fig. 6. Sample plots of joint kinetics and powers for the hip, knee, and ankle in all three cardinal planes of motion. All data are plotted in stance and represent a sample of healthy runners collected at the University of Virginia Center for Endurance Sport Gait Laboratory.

and efficiency may be maintained across a wide variety of terrain.[24] This compensation maintains COM in a somewhat consistent oscillatory path throughout a wide range of real-world conditions, because excessive rise and fall or the excessive minimizing of the COM has been associated with increased energy expenditure.[24]

Ankle, knee, and hip power patterns are similar to those in walking, except that the amplitudes of power absorption and generation are related to the speed (greater power for greater velocity). Ankle patterns are fairly similar to those in walking, with the joint moment speed faster because of shorter contact time and a higher GRF. Knee sagittal moments in running are higher than in walking. In running the knee is more flexed throughout the stance phase, thus requiring more internal muscular support to maintain stability through midstance. Hip sagittal plane moments are similar to those in walking, except the amplitude is greater in running.

Arm movement has been discounted as a source of propulsion in distance running, and said to produce only lift.[43] Conversely, Novacheck and colleagues[44] identifies the arms as aiding a constant horizontal velocity through counterbalancing the rotation of the lower extremity. The upper body is unique in that it shows gross stabilization deficits in the lower body. An excessively wide arm swing can be a strategy to provide additional lateral support when core/hip control is diminished. Excessive crossover of the arms may indicate a lack of stability in the transverse plane. Although these cues do not identify the exact cause of the imbalance, they reveal movement patterns that may be the cause or, conversely, the compensation for the default.

Restricted hip flexors, lumbar spine extensors, thoracodorsal fascia, inadequate core muscle support, chronic low back pain, posture dysfunction, or postural fatigue during a run can move the runner into excessive lumbar spine extension. This extended lumbar spine position can alter forces at the lower extremity, because the COM tends to migrate forward with changes in trunk angle.[45] Observation of the runner "fresh" and also several miles into a run can reveal unique gait traits that affect gross movement pattern dysfunction.

Additional tools can be used to obtain gait parameters: accelerometers allow measure of loading rate of structure, dynamic electromyography allows examination of the respective muscles responsible for internal joint moment, and monitoring oxygen consumption allows data on the metabolic economy of gait to be collected.[46] All gait technologies have their role; the key is to use the technology that can obtain the parameters of interest.

Economy of Motion

Metabolic efficiency is often discussed in terms of physiologic training; however, biomechanical constraints do have a role. Efficiency equals mechanical work/metabolic work. Martin and Morgan[47] identified four primary areas of study: body structure, kinematics, kinetics, and biomechanical feedback/training. However, they were unable to determine how to improve biomechanical economy. Individuals seem to freely choose their most economic speed when walking, as shown by the inverted U theory in **Fig. 7**. Between 1.1 and 1.4 m/s, a relatively flat energy curve range, is observed. Slower speed is more metabolically costly for distance given, whereas excessively fast walking speeds show the same trend. This fact provides evidence that a freely chosen range of walking velocities are optimal. During running, no single range of velocities seems as optimal, in that the faster velocity is offset by additional distance covered. Regarding metabolic economy in running, little correlation exists between the energy invested to cover a given distance and distance travelled. Mechanisms that do affect metabolic economy are believed to include stride length, stride frequency, muscle shortening velocity, and mechanical power output. Kram and

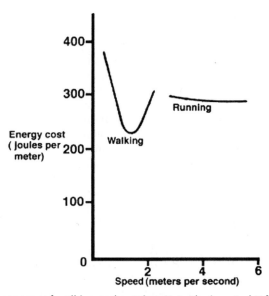

Fig. 7. Metabolic economy of walking and running. Note the inverted *U* for walking and the relatively flat curve for running energy consumption.

Taylor[32] claim the two most important biomechanical constraints in running economy are the total mechanical work done by the body to support the COM in stance, and the inverse relationship with ground contact time (the lower the time of contact, the higher the expenditure).

Current literature supports three critical aspects with respect to biomechanical economy: (1) minimizing the active muscle mass recruited, (2) aligning the legs with the net force vector, and (3) maximizing the effects of elastic recoil. Increased vertical GRF reflects an increase in motor units to go from point *A* to point *B* at a given velocity. Greater force equals greater metabolic cost. Decreased ground contact time minimizes the change in vertical COM height, which in turn increases leg stiffness and causes an increased peak GRF. Optimum ground contact time should be short enough to minimize muscle work but long enough to allow for the release of elastic recoil from the tendons.[32,48] In this manner, the average force production from each leg (the area under the curve) is maximized without increasing the peak force produced. Furthermore, a change in the vertical component is accompanied through a change in the horizontal component (if peak vertical GRF decreases, then acceleration and braking forces also decrease).

Aligning the force vector closer to the leg decreases the external joint moment and minimizes muscle cost.[48] This function is achieved through running with straighter limbs during the stance phase. Using straighter limbs to avoid excessive energy loss with increased joint excursion from flight to stance-phase absorption can help maximize the effects of elastic recoil.[48] Additionally, individualized drills and neuromuscular activities that compliment runners' structure will train them to use elastic recoil in gait. Although sufficient data from multiple works reinforce these concepts, many questions remain unanswered because of the multifactorial and complimentary nature of gait attributes.[49]

Observational gait analysis, although not as specific as 3D analysis, can improve a clinician's ability to bridge the outcome of special tests of dynamic function in gait. The use of slow-motion video capture can vastly improve visualization of gait form. Requirements include a high-quality video camera, a tripod, and video editing software. Video software makes it possible to edit, slow, or freeze-frame footage for specific analysis. Observational video analysis should comprise 30- to 45-second long data collections from multiple angles: front upper body, front lower body, side upper body, side lower body, rear full body, and posterior view from the knee down for a closer look at the foot function. The most important thing is to be consistent when looking at gait; each evaluation should be approached the same each time, irrespective of diagnosis. Often the site of symptom presentation is not the location of biomechanical fault. Altered upper body and trunk movement patterns may reflect alteration in lateral or rotational plane instability. Special attention to the joint above and below the symptom presentation is essential. Through the course of the video evaluation, the observed asymmetry or gait abnormality should be correlated to the clinical examination findings. The goal is to identify a particular biomechanical pattern that could be affecting the individual's symptoms.

Examining individuals dynamically provides a perspective on how they use their combination of strength, flexibility, and muscle memory to achieve gait. Ignoring the biomechanical cause of the imbalance will likely result in the dysfunction becoming adopted into their repetitive gait pattern. Modern gait analysis is a tool to produce objective, quantitative parameters that identify the source of dysfunction in an individual or population. Understanding the concepts behind repetitive loading of running will enable a more directed approach to diagnosis and treatment intervention.

REFERENCES

1. Birrer RB, Buzermanis S, DelaCorte MP, et al. Biomechanics of running. In: O'conor F, Wilder R, editors. The textbook of running medicine. New York: McGraw Hill; 2001. p. 11–9.
2. Dugan SA, Bhat KP. Biomechanics and analysis of running gait [review]. Phys Med Rehabil Clin N Am 2005;16(3):603–21.
3. Novacheck TF. The biomechanics of running. Gait Posture 1998;7:77–95.
4. Kerrigan DC, Edelstein JE. Gait. In: Gonzalez EG, Myers SJ, Edelstein JE, et al, editors. Downey and Darling's physiologic basis of rehabilitation medicine. 3rd edition. Boston: Butterworth-Heineman; 2001. p. 397–416.
5. Kerrigan DC, Della Crose U. Gait analysis. In: O'Connor FG, Sallis RE, Wilder RP, et al, editors. Sports medicine: just the facts. McGraw Hill; 2005. p. 126–30.
6. Gerlach KE, White SC, Burton HW, et al. Kinetic changes with fatigue and relationship to injury in female runners. Med Sci Sports Exerc 2005;37(4):657–63.
7. Della Croce U, Cappozzo A, Kerrigan DC. Pelvic and lower anatomical landmark calibration and its propagation to bone geometry and joint angles. Med Biol Eng Comput 1999;37(2):155–61.
8. Frigo C, Rabuffetti M, Kerrigan DC, et al. Functionally oriented and clinically feasible quantitative gait analysis method. Med Biol Eng Comput 1998;36(2): 179–85.
9. Leardini A, Benedetti MG, Catani F, et al. An anatomical based protocol for the description of foot segment kinematics during gait. Clin Biomech 1999;14: 528–36.
10. Leardini A, Chiari L, Della Croce U, et al. Human movement analysis using stereophotogrammetry, part 3. Soft tissue artifact assessment and compensation. Gait Posture 2005;21:212–25.

11. Nester C, Jones RK, Liu A, et al. Foot kinematics during walking measured using bone and surface mounted markers. J Biomech 2007;40:3412–23.

12. Franz JR, Paylo KW, Dicharry J, et al. Changes in the coordination of hip and pelvis kinematics with mode of locomotion. Gait Posture 2009;29(3):494–8.

13. Hodges PW. Core stability exercise in chronic low back pain. Orthop Clin North Am 2003;34(2):245–54.

14. Chumanov ES, Heiderscheit BC, Thelen DG. The effect of speed and influence of individual muscles on hamstring mechanics during the swing phase of sprinting. J Biomech 2007;40(16):3555–62.

15. Thelen DG, Chumanov ES, Sherry MA, et al. Neuromusculoskeletal models provide insights into the mechanisms and rehabilitation of hamstring strains. Exerc Sport Sci Rev 2006;34(3):135–41.

16. Souza RB, Powers CM. Differences in hip kinematics, muscle strength, and muscle activation between subjects with and without patellofemoral pain. J Orthop Sports Phys Ther 2009;39(1):12–9.

17. Souza RB, Powers CM. Predictors of hip internal rotation during running: an evaluation of hip strength and femoral structure in women with and without patellofemoral pain. Am J Sports Med 2009;37(3):579–87.

18. Leardini A, Benedetti MG, Berti L, et al. Rear-foot, mid-foot, and fore-foot motion during the stance phase of gait. Gait Posture 2007;25:453–62.

19. McPoil T, Cornwall MW. Relationship between neutral subtalar joint position and pattern of rearfoot motion during walking. Foot Ankle Int 1994;15:141–5.

20. Dicharry JM, Franz JR, Della Croce UD, et al. Differences in static and dynamic measures in evaluation of talonavicular mobility in gait. J Orthop Sports Phys Ther 2009;39(8):628–34.

21. Giannini S, Catani F, Benedetti M, et al. Gait analysis: methodologies and clinical applications. Amsterdam: BTS Bioengineering Technology and Systems; 1994.

22. Riley PO, Dicharry J, Franz J, et al. A kinematics and kinetic comparison of overground and treadmill running. Med Sci Sports Exerc 2008;40(6):1093–100.

23. Gottschall JS, Kram R. Ground reaction forces during downhill and uphill running. J Biomech 2005;38(3):445–52.

24. Farley CT, Gonzalez O. Leg stiffness and stride frequency in human running. J Biomech 1996;29(2):181–6.

25. Pope RP. Prevention of pelvic stress fractures in female army recruits. Mil Med 1999;164(5):370–3.

26. Hreljac A, Marshall RN, Hume PA. Evaluation of lower extremity overuse injury potential in runners. Med Sci Sports Exerc 2000;32(9):1635–41.

27. Hreljac A. Impact and overuse injuries in runners. Med Sci Sports Exerc 2004;36(5):845–9.

28. Nigg BM. The role of impact forces and foot pronation: a new paradigm. [review]. Clin J Sport Med 2001;11(1):2–9.

29. O'Connor JA, Lanyon LE. The influence of strain rate on adaptive bone remodeling. J Biomech 1982;15:767–81.

30. Scott SH, Winter DA. Internal forces at chronic running injury sites. Med Sci Sports Exerc 1990;22:357–69.

31. Kerdok AE, Biewener AA, McMahon TA, et al. Energetics and mechanics of human running on surfaces of different stiffnesses. J Appl Physiol 2002;92(2):469–78.

32. Kram R, Taylor CR. Energetics of running: a new perspective. Nature 1990;346(6281):265–7.

33. Wright S, Weyland PS. The application of ground force explains the energetic cost of running backward and forward. J Exp Biol 2001;204:1805–15.

34. Cavanaugh PR, Lafortune MA. Ground reaction forces in distance running. J Biomech 1980;13:397.

35. Mann RA, Hagley J. Biomechanics of walking running, and sprinting. Am J Sports Med 1980;8(5):345–50.

36. Roberts TJ, Marsh RL, Weyand PG, et al. Muscular force in running turkeys: the economy of minimizing work. Science 1997;275(5303):1113–5.

37. Jacobs R, Bobbert MF, van Ingen Schenau GJ. Mechanical output from individual muscles during explosive leg extensions: the role of biarticular muscles. J Biomech 1996;29(4):513–23.

38. Prilutsky BI, Zatsiorsky VM. Tendon action of two joint muscles: transfer of mechanical energy between two joints during jumping, landing, and running. J Biomech 1994;27(1):25–34.

39. Donelan JM, Kram R, Kuo AD. Simultaneous positive and negative external mechanical work in human walking. J Biomech 2002;35:117–24.

40. Donelan JM, Kram R, Kuo AD. Mechanical work for step to step transitions is a major determinant of the metabolic cost of human walking. J Exp Biol 2002; 205:3717–27.

41. Biewener AA, Farley CT, Roberts TJ, et al. Muscle mechanical advantage of human walking and running: implications for energy cost. J Appl Physiol 2004; 97:2266–74.

42. Teunissen L, Grabowski A, Kram R. The effects of independently altering body weight and body mass on the metabolic cost of running. J Exp Biol 2007;210: 4418–27.

43. Hinrichs RN. Upper extremity function in distance running. In: Cavanaugh PR, editor. Biomechanics of distance running. Champaign (IL): Human Kinetics; 1990. p. 107–33.

44. Novacheck TF, Trost JP, Schutte L. Running and sprinting: a dynamic analysis. St Paul (MN): Gillette Children's Hospital; 1996. [Video CD-ROM].

45. Hart JM, Kerrigan DC, Fritz JM, et al. Jogging gait kinetics following fatiguing lumbar paraspinal exercise. J Electromyogr Kinesiol 2009;19(6):e458–64.

46. Perry J. Gait analysis: normal and pathological function. Thorofare (NJ): SLACK; 1992.

47. Martin PE, Morgan DW. Biomechanical considerations for economical walking and running. Med Sci Sports Exerc 1992;24(4):407–74.

48. Chang Y, Huang HC, Hamerski C, et al. The independent effects of gravity and inertia on running mechanics. J Exp Biol 2000;203:229–38.

49. McCann DJ, Higginson BK. Training to maximize economy of motion in running gait. Curr Sports Med Rep 2008;7:158–62.

Flexibility for Runners

Jeffrey Jenkins, MD[a],*, James Beazell, PT, DPT, OCS, ATC[b]

KEYWORDS

• Flexibility • Range of motion • Stretching • PNF

"Flexibility" generally describes the range of motion commonly present in a joint or group of joints that allows normal and unimpaired function.[1] More specifically, flexibility has been defined as the total achievable excursion (within the limits of pain) of a body part through its range of motion.[2] With regard to flexibility, the following generalizations can be made: flexibility is an individually variable, joint-specific, inherited characteristic that decreases with age, varies by gender and ethnic group, bears little relationship with body proportion or limb length, and, most importantly, for the purposes of this article, can be modified through training.[1,3–6]

Achieving a maximal functional range of motion is an important goal of many therapeutic exercise regimens. Most typically, increased range of motion is achieved via the process of stretching. The term "stretching" defines an activity that applies a deforming force along the rotational or translational planes of motion of a joint. Stretching should respect the lines of geometry of the joint and its planes of stability. In addition to stretching, "mobilization" is used to maintain flexibility. Mobilization moves a joint through its range of motion without applying a deforming force.[7]

The athletic literature seems to show that flexibility training, when used appropriately, plays a positive role in sports injury and performance. However, excessive flexibility may actually be both a risk factor for injury[5,8–11] and a detriment to performance. Stiff structures do seem to benefit from stretching, whereas hypermobile structures require stabilization rather than additional mobilization.

DETERMINANTS OF FLEXIBILITY

The determinants of joint mobility can be subdivided into static and dynamic factors. Static factors include the types of tissues involved, the state of collagen subunits in the tissue, the presence or absence of inflammation, and the temperature of the tissue. Dynamic factors include neuromuscular variables such as voluntary muscle control

[a] Department of Physical Medicine and Rehabilitation, University of Virginia, 545 Ray C. Hunt Drive, Suite 240, Charlottesville, VA 22903, USA
[b] University of Virginia–HealthSouth Physical Therapy, 545 Ray C. Hunt Drive, Suit 210, Charlottesville, VA 22903, USA
* Corresponding author.
E-mail address: jj5u@virginia.edu

Clin Sports Med 29 (2010) 365–377
doi:10.1016/j.csm.2010.03.004
0278-5919/10/$ – see front matter © 2010 Elsevier Inc. All rights reserved.

and the inherent neuromuscular feedback of the musculotendinous unit, as well as external factors such as pain associated with injury.[2]

Static Factors

The most important tissue with regard to flexibility is the muscle-tendon unit (MTU), which is the primary target of flexibility training.[2] This structure includes the full length of the muscle and its supporting tissue, the musculotendinous junction, and the full length of the tendon to the tendon-bone junction. The MTU has both viscous and elastic mechanical properties. The MTU reacts to a slowly applied stretching force with elongation, a phenomenon called stress relaxation. This phenomenon is accomplished through the mechanical property of creep. The viscous aspect of the MTU means that rapidly applied force to the muscle will be met by increased resistance to elongation.

Within the MTU, it is the muscle that has the largest capacity for percent lengthening[12–14] of the tissues involved in a stretch. A ratio of 95%:5% for muscle:tendon length change has been demonstrated.[14] From a mechanical standpoint, muscle is composed of contractile and series elastic elements arranged in parallel.[15] Muscle can respond to an applied force or stretch with permanent elongation. Animal studies have shown that this results from an increase in the number of sarcomeres, which translates to increased peak tension of a muscle at longer resting lengths. By contrast, muscle at rest has a tendency to shorten because of its contractile element. This shortening can be permanent and is associated with a reduction in sarcomeres.[16–19] Tendon has a much more limited capacity for lengthening than muscle, probably because of its proteoglycan content and collagen cross-links (2%–3% of its length, compared with 20% for muscle).[13,14,18] Of the external static factors, temperature has been studied the most. Warmer tissues are generally more distensible than colder ones.[19–21]

Dynamic Factors

Perhaps the most clinically and physiologically significant dynamic determinant of flexibility is the muscle length-tension thermostat or feedback control system. Intrafusal fibers (muscle spindles), innervated by gamma motoneurons, lie in parallel with extrafusal contractile fibers. The intrafusal fibers serve the purpose of regulating the tension and length of the muscle as a whole. Muscle spindle length and tension are regulated by the gamma motoneuron, which in turn is subject to influences from the central nervous system. These include segmental input at the spinal cord level and suprasegmental input from the cerebellum and cortex. Consequently, muscle length and tension can be subject to multiple influences simultaneously. An additional complicating factor is that receptors in the musculotendinous unit called the Golgi tendon organs (GTOs) act to inhibit muscle contraction at the point of critical stresses to the structure. The GTOs allow lengthening and facilitate relaxation. When acting in conjunction, these dynamic mechanisms facilitate a response to a stretch in the following ways: as the muscle spindle is initially stretched, it sends impulses to the spinal cord that result in reflex muscle contraction, and if the stretch is maintained longer than 6 seconds, the GTO fires, causing relaxation.[2] The relative contribution of static muscle factors and dynamic neural factors to flexibility remains somewhat controversial. The changes in flexibility noted immediately after the institution of a stretching program occur too rapidly to be attributable solely to structural alteration of the muscle and connective tissue. The consensus view is that neural factors probably play the major role in this early flexibility. After prolonged periods of training, changes in sarcomere number can play a role in the establishment of a new elongated muscle length.[2]

ASSESSMENT OF FLEXIBILITY

Flexibility is generally assessed in terms of joint range of motion. Joint range of motion in turn is generally assessed with a goniometer or a similar device. A goniometer consists of a 180° protractor that is designed for easy application to joints. The methods used when using a goniometer, as well as the normal ranges of motion encountered with these methods, are well standardized.[22] Inter- and intra-observer reliabilities are good.[8] Limitations of the standard goniometer include application to only single joints at a given time, static measurements only, and difficulty of application to certain joints (eg, costoclavicular joint). The Leighton Flexometer (Leighton Flexometer, Inc, Spokane, WA, USA) contains a rotating circular dial marked in degrees and a pointer counterbalanced to remain vertical. It can be strapped to a body segment, and range of motion is determined with respect to the perpendicular. Leighton Flexometer's reliability is good but is not equivalent to that of the standard goniometer.[23] The electrogoniometer substitutes a potentiometer for a protractor. The potentiometer provides an electrical signal that is directly proportional to the angle of the joint. This device is able to give continuous recordings during a variety of activities, allowing a more realistic assessment of functional flexibility and dynamic range of motion during actual physical activity.

METHODS OF STRETCHING

It is important to take several factors into consideration when using a stretching program. Prevention of injury and treatment of specific joint injury, as well as the presence and effects of pain or muscle spasm, require modification of the program. Stretching can be dangerous and might result in significant injury if performed incorrectly.[24–26] As with any form of therapeutic exercise, flexibility training must be approached within a program aimed at addressing the specific functional needs of the individual. Numerous options are now available for improving flexibility with stretching techniques. A distinct superiority of any 1 method has not been demonstrated. For the purposes of this article, stretching techniques are divided into the following 4 categories: ballistic, static, passive, and proprioceptive neuromuscular facilitation (PNF).

Ballistic Stretching

Ballistic stretching uses the repetitive rapid application of force in a bouncing or jerking maneuver. Momentum carries the body part through the range of motion until the muscles are stretched to the limits. This method is less efficient than other methods as the muscle will contract under these stresses to protect itself from overstretching. In addition, the rapid increase in force can cause injury.[25,27] An example would be the 10-count bouncing toe touches popularized in the 1970s but since abandoned because of perceived lack of efficacy and documented risk of injury. Recent evidence has begun to revive interest in this recently disparaged form of flexibility training. Witvrouw and colleagues[28] have reported that ballistic stretching may have beneficial effects on tendon elasticity. They propose that this effect may be important in athletes who perform more jumping activities, which are considered stretch-shortening cycles. The stretch-shortening phenomenon is important in absorbing force and then saving it as potential energy. The theory is that ballistic stretching may activate the muscle to a significantly greater degree than static stretching, resulting in a significantly greater load on the corresponding tendon and bringing about an improvement in its elasticity.

Passive Stretching

Passive stretching uses a partner or therapist who applies a stretch to a relaxed joint or extremity. This method requires excellent communication and the slow and sensitive application of force. This method is most appropriately and most safely used in the training room or in a physical or occupational therapy context. Outside these contexts, passive stretching can be dangerous for recreational or competitive athletes because of increased risk of injury. In their 2005 study, Verrall and colleagues[29] successfully incorporated a passive hamstring stretching program into an overall training program for an Australian rules football team. They were able to show a significant decrease in hamstring strains per 1000 hours of playing time in their subjects.

Static Stretching

Static stretching applies a steady force for a period of 15 to 60 seconds. This method is the easiest, certainly is the most popular, and may be the safest type of stretching. Perhaps consequently, static stretching is also the most studied form of flexibility training. Since the early eighties, static stretching has been encouraged as a warm-up activity before any other form of therapeutic or recreational exercise, including athletic activity. Static stretching has the added advantage here of being associated with decreased muscle soreness after exercise.[30,31] This advantage may contribute to its efficacy. Bjorklund and colleagues[32] showed that sensory adaptation seems to be an important mechanistic factor in the effect stretching has on range of motion changes.

In a systematic review of static stretching as warm-up to prevent injury, Small and colleagues[33] were able to find only 4 randomized controlled trials and 3 clinical controlled trials that were of high enough quality to include. The investigators concluded that there is moderate to strong evidence to indicate that static stretching does not reduce overall injury rates. However, they did suggest that there is preliminary evidence that static stretching may specifically reduce musculotendinous injuries. This finding was based primarily on the conclusions of 2 articles, specifically those by Amako and colleagues[34] and Bixler and Jones.[35] Both of these studies were able to show a significant reduction in musculotendinous injuries after implementation of a static stretching program, whereas neither found a significant difference in overall injury rate. Another review article by Woods and colleagues[36] in 2007 also cited the work of Amako, Bixler, and Jones, but in addition, referenced the findings of Hartig and Henderson[37] and Verrall and colleagues[29] This review was more positive regarding the effects of flexibility training and concluded that stretching programs have consistently shown a positive effect on the prevention of muscular injury.

The neural effects of static stretching[38] have been studied in the soleus muscle, and the effect on the muscle spindle has been studied by observing changes in the Hoffmann reflex (H-reflex) and tendon reflex (T-reflex). The results indicated that the H-reflex decreased significantly more than the T-reflex during progressive stretching. Both the H- and T-reflexes stay depressed during the stretch, and the H-reflex returns to normal after the stretch is removed, whereas the T-reflex remains below the control value. The conclusion is that the resultant inhibition of the T-reflex is the result of either decreased muscle spindle sensitivity or increased compliance of the MTU.

PROPRIOCEPTIVE NEUROMUSCULAR FACILITATION

PNF has been a component of specific training of patients with neuromuscular disease or injury. PNF was developed by Kabat and Knott[39] and based on the neuromuscular concepts developed by Sherrington and Laslett's research[40] at the beginning of the 20th century. In an excellent review of the research on PNF stretching, Sharman and colleagues[41] describe the current theories on the physiologic mechanisms that are responsible for the effectiveness of PNF training.

Sharman and colleagues[41] found that PNF techniques and descriptions of those techniques were highly variable, making it difficult to compare various studies. However, there is general consensus that the effectiveness of PNF stretching is based on neurophysiologic effects. Two specific mechanisms are theorized to mediate this response: autogenic inhibition and reciprocal inhibition.

Autogenic inhibition is theorized to be due to the stretch of GTOs in the MTU, resulting in a decrease in the muscle excitability after stretching. This muscle excitability would allow for the elongation of the muscle after inhibition as a result of activation of the GTO. Research has failed to prove this theory on a consistent basis, and this effect has been shown only to last at most 1 second after the contraction has ended.[42]

Reciprocal inhibition refers to the effect of contraction of the opposing muscle on the muscle targeted for stretching. This proposed mechanism holds that efferent input into the spinal cord will alter the presynaptic inhibition of the muscle to be stretched. Specifically, descending motor input activates not only alpha motoneurons to the opposing muscle but also the inhibitory 1a afferent neurons of the target muscle to be stretched. Evidence for this mechanism is mixed. On the one hand, research has not shown a difference in motoneuron pool excitability between static stretching and PNF stretching[42] as reflected in either electromyography or H-reflex recordings. However, few studies have shown that contraction of the opposing muscle to the target muscle for stretching does cause a greater increase in range of motion.[41]

ATHLETIC PERFORMANCE

In addition to injury prevention, another proposed benefit of flexibility training is improved sports performance. With regard to running, the evidence for this effect is weak at best. Several laboratories have shown that among runners, less-flexible individuals have a lower rate of oxygen consumption while covering the same distance at the same speed as their more flexible cohorts.[4,43] In addition, the in vitro improvement in contraction strength resulting from prestretching[44–47] has not been consistently observed in the world of athletics. It has been shown repeatedly that passive stretching can result in an acute loss of strength.[48–53] Along the same lines, a recent study of elite female soccer players demonstrated that static stretching before sprinting resulted in worsened performance.[54] Stretching too vigorously before an athletic event is likely to impair performance. The injury prevention role of stretching has to be balanced against this consideration on an individual athlete-to-athlete basis.

FLEXIBILITY PROGRAM

Runners are likely to benefit from a flexibility program. Various stretches have been espoused for the muscles of the lower quarter. What follows is the flexibility program developed at the Runner's Clinic at the University of Virginia.

Hip Flexors

Effects of hip flexor stretching have been studied in elderly with gait. Subjects performing a home program of hip flexor stretching improved their hip extension

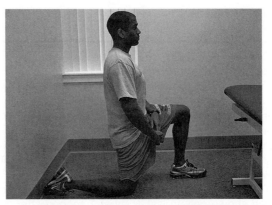

Fig. 1. Hip flexor stretch. Athlete is in 90/90 position. Perform a posterior pelvic tilt to activate the right gluteal as shown to facilitate stretch of iliopsoas. Avoid lumbar extension or passive hip extension. Stretch should be vaguely felt in anterior thigh.

compared with control subjects who are at both self-selected gait speed and fast walking.[55] A stretch using the PNF concept of reciprocal inhibition can be performed as shown in **Fig. 1**. In this position, the athlete performs a posterior pelvic tilt while contracting the gluteals that will facilitate a stretch of the iliopsoas complex.

Hamstrings

A systematic review was performed in 2005[56] to determine the most appropriate hamstring stretch technique and duration. The investigators concluded that various techniques improved flexibility with various durations of application of the stretch and different positions. A randomized controlled trial[57] comparing 4 different stretching techniques in a cohort of 100 subjects showed that active stretch using a reciprocal inhibition contraction of the quadriceps (**Fig. 2**) and passive straight leg raise (**Fig. 3**) improved hamstring flexibility.

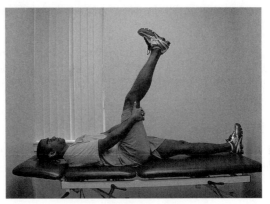

Fig. 2. Active hamstring stretch. Athlete flexes hip up to 90° and clasps behind knee. Athlete then attempts to straighten knee to activate quadriceps and stretch hamstrings. The athlete can increase the hip flexion to change stretch emphasis.

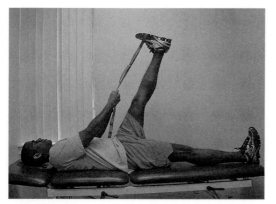

Fig. 3. Passive hamstring stretch.

Quadriceps

A simple stretching program of the quadriceps (**Fig. 4**) has been shown to be effective and associated with some decrease in pain in patients with patellofemoral pain.[58] The investigators reported significant change in Kendall test (**Fig. 5**) for quadriceps length and associated improvement in pain and function.

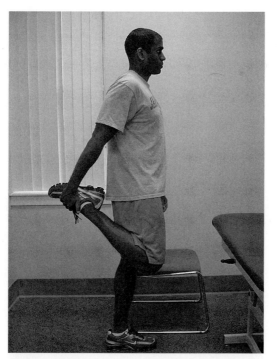

Fig. 4. Quadriceps stretch. Keeping the trunk, hip, and knee in alignment, the athlete bends the knee and grasps with the ipsilateral hand; the contralateral hand can grasp a chair for balance. The stretch can be accentuated with bending of the stance knee.

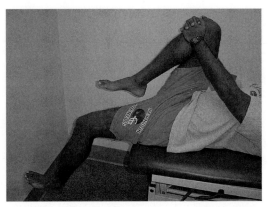

Fig. 5. Kendall test for quadriceps length. The angle of the knee is measured with the athlete in the Thomas test position.

Rectus Femoris

Isolated rectus femoris stretching can be performed in prone with the opposite leg in hip flexion off a treatment table. The athlete maintains their lumbar spine in neutral and can use a belt to flex the knee. An anterior pelvic tilt can be performed to increase the stretch of the rectus femoris (**Fig. 6**).

Iliotibial Band

Fredericson and colleagues[59] evaluated a series of stretches that focused on the iliotibial band (ITB) in 5 asymptomatic runners in a biomechanics laboratory. All 3 stretches (**Fig. 7**) were statistically significant in increasing the stretch in the ITB, hip adduction, and knee adduction moments. To perform the standing stretch, the athlete stands upright, using a wall for balance if needed. The leg to be stretched is extended and adducted behind the uninvolved leg. The athlete side bends to the opposite side until a stretch is felt laterally on the hip. The athlete can tilt the pelvis to change the area

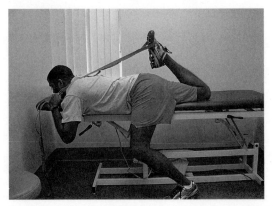

Fig. 6. Rectus femoris stretch. Athlete stabilizes pelvis with left leg off table and uses belt to stretch right rectus femoris.

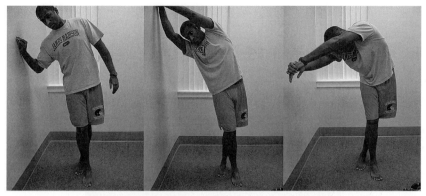

Fig. 7. Iliotibial band stretch. The athlete stands upright, using a wall for balance if needed. The leg to be stretched is extended and adducted behind the uninvolved leg. The athlete side bends to the opposite side until a stretch is felt laterally on the hip. The athlete can tilt the pelvis to change the area of stretch. The arm can be reached overhead, and the stretch of the hip can be accentuated by increasing the side bending of the trunk.

of stretch. The arm can be reached overhead and the stretch of the hip can be accentuated by increasing the side bending of the trunk.

Gastrocnemius

Flexibility of the gastrocsoleus complex is important to allow forward translation of the tibia during the stance phase of walking and running. Clinically, making sure that the athlete is maintaining a neutral subtalar joint position to not contribute to an excessive pronation strategy to compensate for a restricted gastrocsoleus muscle flexibility, perform with the knee bent as well as straight (**Fig. 8**).

Toe Flexors/Plantar Fascia

Stretching of the plantar fascia has been reported to be effective in patients with acute plantar fasciitis. The athlete is instructed to sit with the leg of the foot to be stretched crossed over the opposite leg and the hand grasping the toes to flex them until a stretch is felt in the bottom of the foot (**Fig. 9**).

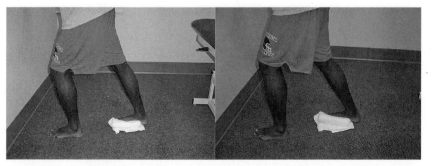

Fig. 8. Gastrocnemius/soleus stretch. A towel can be placed under the medial arch to help maintain subtalar neutral, and the knee can track over the second toe to effective stretch this muscle group.

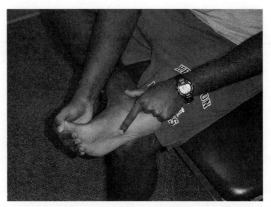

Fig. 9. Plantar fascia stretch. The leg is crossed over the opposite leg. The ipsilateral hand extends the toes, and the contralateral hand can monitor the stretch in the plantar fascia.

SUMMARY

The literature on flexibility presents the evidence-based practitioner with some basic science information, a good background on the mechanisms of proposed methods of flexibility training, as well as varied results as to the effectiveness of these programs. A general overview of flexibility and its components as well as the authors' flexibility program at the Runner's Clinic at the University of Virginia has been presented. As stated in one review, methodological disparities and inconsistencies make analyzing the flexibility literature difficult and confusing.

REFERENCES

1. Corbin CB. Flexibility. Clin Sports Med 1984;3:101–17.
2. Saal J. Flexibility taining. In: Kibler W, editor. Functional rehabilitation of sports and musculoskeletal injuries. Gaithersburg (MD): Aspen; 1998. p. 85–97.
3. Gleim GW, McHugh MP. Flexibility and its effects on sports injury and performance. Sports Med 1997;24:289–99.
4. Grahame R, Jenkins JM. Joint hypermobility–asset or liability? A study of joint mobility in ballet dancers. Ann Rheum Dis 1972;31:109–11.
5. Grahame R. Joint hypermobility–clinical aspects. Proc R Soc Med 1971;64:692–4.
6. Grana WA, Moretz JA. Ligamentous laxity in secondary school athletes. JAMA 1978;240:1975–6.
7. Wilder RP, Jenkins J, Seto C. Therapeutic exercise. In: Braddom R, editor. Physical medicine and rehabilitation. Philadelphia: Elsevier; 2007. p. 413–36.
8. Ekstrand J, Gillquist J. The avoidability of soccer injuries. Int J Sports Med 1983;4:124–8.
9. Godshall RW. The predictability of athletic injuries: an eight-year study. J Sports Med 1975;3:50–4.
10. Keller CS, Noyes FR, Buncher CR. The medical aspects of soccer injury epidemiology. Am J Sports Med 1987;15:230–7.
11. Lysens RJ, Ostyn MS, Vanden Auweele Y, et al. The accident-prone and overuse-prone profiles of the young athlete. Am J Sports Med 1989;17:612–9.

12. Johns R, Wright V. Relative importance of various tissues in joint stiffness. J Appl Physiol 1962;17:814–28.
13. Stolov WC, Fry LR, Riddell WM, et al. Adhesive forces between muscle fibers and connective tissue in normal and denervated rat skeletal muscle. Arch Phys Med Rehabil 1973;54:208–13.
14. Stolov WC, Weilepp TG Jr. Passive length-tension relationship of intact muscle, epimysium, and tendon in normal and denervated gastrocnemius of the rat. Arch Phys Med Rehabil 1966;47:612–20.
15. Huxley AF, Simmons RM. Mechanical properties of the cross-bridges of frog striated muscle. J Physiol 1971;218:59P–60P.
16. Goldspink DF. The influence of immobilization and stretch on protein turnover of rat skeletal muscle. J Physiol 1977;264:267–82.
17. Goldspink DF, Williams P. The nature of the increased passive resitance in muscle following immobilization of the mouse soleus muscle. J Physiol 1979;289:55.
18. Williams PE, Goldspink G. Changes in sarcomere length and physiological properties in immobilized muscle. J Anat 1978;127:459–68.
19. East J, Smith F, Burry L. Evaluation of warm-up for improvement in flexibility. Am J Phys Med 1986;14:316–9.
20. Warren CG, Lehmann JF, Koblanski JN. Heat and stretch procedures: an evaluation using rat tail tendon. Arch Phys Med Rehabil 1976;57:122–6.
21. Wiktorsson-Moller M, Oberg B, Ekstrand J, et al. Effects of warming up, massage, and stretching on range of motion and muscle strength in the lower extremity. Am J Sports Med 1983;11:249–52.
22. Polley H, Hunder G. Physical examination of the joints. Philadelphia: Saunders; 1978.
23. Harris ML. Flexibility. Phys Ther 1969;49:591–601.
24. Sady SP, Wortman M, Blanke D. Flexibility training: ballistic, static or proprioceptive neuromuscular facilitation? Arch Phys Med Rehabil 1982;63:261–3.
25. Shellock FG, Prentice WE. Warming-up and stretching for improved physical performance and prevention of sports-related injuries. Sports Med 1985;2:267–78.
26. Shyne K, Dominquez R. To stretch or not to stretch. Phys Sports Med 1982;10:137–40.
27. Surburg P. Flexibility exercises re-examined. J Athl Train 1983;18:370–4.
28. Witvrouw E, Mahieu N, Roosen P, et al. The role of stretching in tendon injuries. Br J Sports Med 2007;41:224–6.
29. Verrall GM, Slavotinek JP, Barnes PG. The effect of sports specific training on reducing the incidence of hamstring injuries in professional Australian rules football players. Br J Sports Med 2005;39:363–8.
30. DeVries H. Electromyographic observations of effects of static stretching upon muscular distress. Res Q 1960;32:468–79.
31. deVries HA. Prevention of muscular distress after exercises. Res Q 1960;32:177–85.
32. Bjorklund M, Hamberg J, Crenshaw AG. Sensory adaptation after a 2-week stretching regimen of the rectus femoris muscle. Arch Phys Med Rehabil 2001;82:1245–50.
33. Small K, Mc NL, Matthews M. A systematic review into the efficacy of static stretching as part of a warm-up for the prevention of exercise-related injury. Res Sports Med 2008;16:213–31.
34. Amako M, Oda T, Masuoka K, et al. Effect of static stretching on prevention of injuries for military recruits. Mil Med 2003;168:442–6.

35. Bixler B, Jones RL. High-school football injuries: effects of a post-halftime warm-up and stretching routine. Fam Pract Res J 1992;12:131–9.

36. Woods K, Bishop P, Jones E. Warm-up and stretching in the prevention of muscular injury. Sports Med 2007;37:1089–99.

37. Hartig DE, Henderson JM. Increasing hamstring flexibility decreases lower extremity overuse injuries in military basic trainees. Am J Sports Med 1999;27:173–6.

38. Guissard N, Duchateau J. Neural aspects of muscle stretching. Exerc Sport Sci Rev 2006;34:154–8.

39. Kabat H, Knott M. Principles of neuromuscular reeducation. Phys Ther Rev 1948;28:107–11.

40. Sherrington CS, Laslett EE. Observations on some spinal reflexes and the interconnection of spinal segments. J Physiol 1903;29:58–96.

41. Sharman MJ, Cresswell AG, Riek S. Proprioceptive neuromuscular facilitation stretching: mechanisms and clinical implications. Sports Med 2006;36:929–39.

42. Chalmers G. Re-examination of the possible role of Golgi tendon organ and muscle spindle reflexes in proprioceptive neuromuscular facilitation muscle stretching. Sports Biomech 2004;3:159–83.

43. Gollnick PD, Karlsson J, Piehl K, et al. Selective glycogen depletion in skeletal muscle fibers of man following sustained contractions. J Physiol 1974;241:59–67.

44. Bosco C, Tihanyi J, Komi PV, et al. Store and recoil of elastic energy in slow and fast types of human skeletal muscles. Acta Physiol Scand 1982;116:343–9.

45. Bosco C, Komi PV. Potentiation of the mechanical behavior of the human skeletal muscle through prestretching. Acta Physiol Scand 1979;106:467–72.

46. Cavagna GA, Dusman B, Margaria R. Positive work done by a previously stretched muscle. J Appl Physiol 1968;24:21–32.

47. Cavagna GA, Saibene FP, Margaria R. Effect of negative work on the amount of positive work performed by an isolated muscle. J Appl Physiol 1965;20:157–8.

48. Cramer JT, Housh TJ, Johnson GO, et al. Acute effects of static stretching on peak torque in women. J Strength Cond Res 2004;18:236–41.

49. Cramer JT, Housh TJ, Coburn JW, et al. Acute effects of static stretching on maximal eccentric torque production in women. J Strength Cond Res 2006;20:354–8.

50. Evetovich TK, Nauman NJ, Conley DS, et al. Effect of static stretching of the biceps brachii on torque, electromyography, and mechanomyography during concentric isokinetic muscle actions. J Strength Cond Res 2003;17:484–8.

51. Fowles JR, Sale DG, MacDougall JD. Reduced strength after passive stretch of the human plantarflexors. J Appl Physiol 2000;89:1179–88.

52. Kokkonen J, Nelson AG, Cornwell A. Acute muscle stretching inhibits maximal strength performance. Res Q Exerc Sport 1998;69:411–5.

53. Marek SM, Cramer JT, Fincher AL, et al. Acute effects of static and proprioceptive neuromuscular facilitation stretching on muscle strength and power output. J Athl Train 2005;40:94–103.

54. Sayers AL, Farley RS, Fuller DK, et al. The effect of static stretching on phases of sprint performance in elite soccer players. J Strength Cond Res 2008;22:1416–21.

55. Kerrigan DC, Xenopoulos-Oddsson A, Sullivan MJ, et al. Effect of a hip flexor-stretching program on gait in the elderly. Arch Phys Med Rehabil 2003;84:1–6.

56. Decoster LC, Cleland J, Altieri C, et al. The effects of hamstring stretching on range of motion: a systematic literature review. J Orthop Sports Phys Ther 2005;35:377–87.

57. Fasen JM, O'Connor AM, Schwartz SL, et al. A randomized controlled trial of hamstring stretching: comparison of four techniques. J Strength Cond Res 2009;23:660–7.

58. Peeler J, Anderson JE. Effectiveness of static quadriceps stretching in individuals with patellofemoral joint pain. Clin J Sport Med 2007;17:234–41.

59. Fredericson M, White JJ, Macmahon JM, et al. Quantitative analysis of the relative effectiveness of 3 iliotibial band stretches. Arch Phys Med Rehabil 2002;83: 589–92.

Patellofemoral Pain Syndrome

Hervé Collado, MD[a,b,c],*, Michael Fredericson, MD[d,e,f]

> **KEYWORDS**
> • Patellofemoral • Pain • Syndrome

The average recreational runner has a 37% to 56% incidence of being injured during the course of a year's training.[1] The knee is the most common site of injury and patellofemoral pain (PFP) syndrome constitutes nearly 25% of injuries to the knee.[2] The cause of PFP, however, is not clearly understood and may have multiple origins. The most commonly accepted hypothesis is related to increased patellofemoral joint stress (force per unit area) and subsequent articular cartilage wear.

CLASSIFICATION SYSTEMS

There are many classification systems for PFP. Most of these are based on radiographic findings and grading of the extent of chondral injury or patellar position. These systems are devised to help in surgical planning, but are not easily applicable in the clinical setting. An innovative classification system by Holmes and Clancy[3] (**Box 1**) allows classification of the various patellofemoral pathologies seen in a runner's injury clinic, and particularly in clarifying PFP or instability related to malalignment.

PREDISPOSING FACTORS FOR PATELLAR MALALIGNMENT AND INSTABILITY
Bony Abnormalities

As the knee begins to flex, the articular surface of the patella comes into contact with the lateral femoral condyle and the patella then follows an S-shaped curve through the

[a] Department of Medicine & Rehabilitation and Sport Medicine, University Hospital la Timone, Boulevard Jean Moulin, 13005 Marseille, France
[b] Division of Physical Medicine & Rehabilitation, Stanford University School of Medicine, Stanford, CA, USA
[c] Department of Orthopaedic Surgery, PM&R and Sports Medicine, Stanford University School of Medicine, Stanford, CA, USA
[d] Orthopaedics & Sports Medicine, Stanford University School of Medicine, Stanford Center for Medicine, 450 Broadway Street, Redwood City, CA 94063, USA
[e] PM&R Sports Medicine Service, Stanford University School of Medicine, Stanford Center for Medicine, 450 Broadway Street, Redwood City, CA 94063, USA
[f] Stanford Cross-Country & Track, Stanford University School of Medicine, Stanford Center for Medicine, 450 Broadway Street, Redwood City, CA 94063, USA
* Corresponding author. Department of Medicine & Rehabilitation and Sport Medicine, University Hospital la Timone, Boulevard Jean Moulin, 13005 Marseille, France.
E-mail address: herve.collado@ap-hm.fr

Clin Sports Med 29 (2010) 379–398
doi:10.1016/j.csm.2010.03.012
0278-5919/10/$ – see front matter © 2010 Elsevier Inc. All rights reserved.

sportsmed.theclinics.com

Box 1
Classification of Patellofemoral Pain and Dysfunction

Patellofemoral instability

1. Subluxation or dislocation, single episode
2. Subluxation or dislocation, recurrent
   - Lateral subluxation or dislocation
     Normal functional Q-angle
     Increased functional Q-angle
     Dysplastic trochlea
     Grossly inadequate medial stabilizers
     Patella alta
     Tight lateral retinaculum
   - Medial subluxation or dislocation
     Iatrogenic
3. Chronic dislocation of patella
   - Congenital
   - Acquired
4. Associated fractures
   - Osteochondral
   - Avulsion

Patellofemoral pain and malalignment

1. Increased functional Q-angle
   - Femoral anteversion
   - External tibial torsion
   - Genu valgum
   - Foot hyperpronation
2. Tight lateral retinaculum (lateral patellar compression syndrome)
3. Grossly inadequate medial stabilizers
4. Electrical dissociation
5. Patella alta
6. Patella baja
7. Dysplastic femoral trochlea

Patellofemoral pain without malalignment

1. Tight medial and lateral retinacula
2. Plica
3. Osteochondritis dissecans
   - Patella
   - Femoral trochlea
4. Traumatic patellar chondromalacia
5. Fat pad syndrome

6. Patellofemoral osteoarthritis
   - Posttraumatic
   - Idiopathic
7. Patellar tendinitis
8. Quadriceps tendinitis
9. Prepatellar bursitis
10. Apophysitis
    - Osgood-Schlatter syndrome
    - Sinding-Larsen-Johanssen disease
11. Symptomatic bipartite patella
12. Other trauma
    - Quadriceps tendon rupture
    - Patellar tendon rupture
    - Patella fracture
    - Proximal tibial epiphysis (tubercle) fracture
    - Contusion
    - Turf knee/wrestler's knee
    - Cruciate ligament instability
13. Reflex sympathetic dystrophy

From Holmes WS, Clancy WG. Clinical classification of patellofemoral pain and dysfunction. J Orthop Sports Phys Ther 1998;28(5):300; with permission.

trochlea. Part of the patellar surface remains in contact with the trochlea throughout the remainder of the flexion arc. This contact between the femur and patella progresses from a distal to a proximal direction on the patella.[4] Helping to keep the patella centered in the trochlear groove is the V-shaped anatomy of the patella and the configuration of the femoral condyles. In normal knees the lateral condyle is higher than the medial one. There may be various degrees of true dysplasia of the medial or lateral portions of the trochlear groove, leading to decreased stability of the patellofemoral joint.[5] This instability can be caused by either excessive thickness of the floor of the trochlea or insufficient height of one or both trochlear femoral condyles. Asymmetry of patellar facets also affects patellar congruity. The normal ratio of the lateral to medial facet is 3:2, such that the lateral facet is longer and more sloped, matching the higher and wider lateral femoral condyle.[6]

Lower Extremity Malalignment

Torsional or angular malalignment of the lower extremity has a significant influence on the patellofemoral joint mechanics. Significant deviations in patella alignment secondary to patella alta, trochlear dysplasia, femoral anteversion, knee valgus, and a laterally displaced tibial tuberosity could cause PFP.[7] For example, anteversion of the femoral neck is frequently associated with external torsion of the tibia and, frequently, compensatory pronation of the foot. Hyperpronation of the foot is a causative factor for PFP syndrome (PFPS).[8] In theory, increased pronation causes the tibia to internally rotate during the weight acceptance phase of gait, thereby preventing the tibia from fully externally rotating during midstance. In turn, this prevents the knee from fully locking via the screw-home mechanism. To compensate, the femur internally rotates to allow the knee to fully lock. Increased femoral internal rotation leads to increased contact pressure between the patella and the lateral trochlear groove, which can increase subchondral bone stress and symptoms of PFPS.

Muscle and Soft Tissue Imbalances

One of the most important anatomic factors proposed for affecting dynamic patellar stabilization is the balance between the medial and lateral quadriceps muscles. It is thought that the vastus medialis obliquus (VMO), the primary active medial stabilizer of the patella,[9] is often overpowered by the lateral forces acting on the patella, which include the iliotibial tract, the lateral retinaculum, and the vastus lateralis.[10] In some runners the VMO is weak; however, many runners with sufficient VMO strength still exhibit timing deficit with delayed onset of the VMO when compared with the vastus lateralis.[11,12]

Abnormal soft tissue length can also affect patellofemoral mechanics. For example, tightness in the quadriceps muscle can directly increase the contact pressure between the articular surfaces of the femur and patella, whereas tightness in the hamstrings and gastrocnemius can indirectly increase patellofemoral joint reaction forces by producing a constant flexion moment to the patella.[13] Tightness in the hamstrings or gastrocnemius will also restrict talocrural dorsiflexion, producing compensatory pronation in the subtalar joint[14] and an increase in the dynamic Q-angle. The talocrural joint requires 10° of dorsiflexion for walking and 15° to 25° of dorsiflexion for running. If this motion is not available, compensatory pronation occurs to allow dorsiflexion of the midfoot on the rearfoot.[15]

Tightness of the iliotibial band (ITB) can affect normal patella excursion. The distal ITB fibers blend with the superficial and deep fibers of the lateral retinaculum, and tightness in the ITB can contribute to lateral patellar tilt and excessive pressure on the lateral patella.[7] There is an association between patellar hypomobility and a tight ITB. Hypermobility with increased lateral patellar glide is correlated with laxity of the medial patellofemoral ligament or patellomeniscal ligament, and is often noted in association with patellar subluxation or dislocation.

PATHOPHYSIOLOGY

The pathophysiology of PFP is not well understood. Studies of the biomechanical factors that potentially contribute to PFPS demonstrate conflicting results, a lack of reproducibility, and no firm conclusions. Investigators consistently cite the difficulty of research due to the syndrome's probable multifactorial nature. Proper tracking requires balanced forces acting on the patella. If any force acting on the patella is too large or too small then the movement of the patella may be altered, thereby placing additional stresses on the soft tissue of the joint. As the stress exceeds the tissues' mechanical strength, microdamage, inflammation, and pain result.[16] Altered stresses in the cartilage may also play a role in a pain response by transferring stresses into the underlying subchondral bone and exciting nociceptors. Increased cartilage and subchondral bone stress have been postulated as mechanical causes for PFP,[17] supported, in part, by estimates of average joint stresses (force/area) in patients with PFP.[18] The lateral retinaculum also plays an important role in PFP. The chronic lateral subluxation of the patella can lead to shortening of the retinaculum with secondary nerve damage, resembling the histopathologic picture of a Morton neuroma.[13,19] The synovium, medial patellofemoral ligament, and fat pad of Hoffa, along with the loss of tissue homeostasis, have also been highlighted as potent sources of pain.[20,21]

CLINICAL PRESENTATION

Runners note the insidious onset of an ill-defined ache localized to the anterior knee, behind the knee cap. The onset of anterior knee pain may be gradual or acute and may be precipitated by trauma. Pain may occur in one or both knees. Knee pain worsens with squatting, running, prolonged sitting, or when ascending or descending steps.[22] The pain is often poorly localized under or around the patella, and is usually described as "achy" but may be "sharp." The pain may vary throughout the run and is particularly aggravated by hills. Some patients may describe the affected knee as "giving way" or "buckling." In PFPS this perceived instability may be due to pain inhibiting proper contraction of the quadriceps; but it must be distinguished from instability arising from a patellar dislocation, subluxation, or ligamentous injury of the knee. There may be occasional complaints of mild swelling but it is rare for there to be a gross effusion seen with a traumatic knee injury. In the subset of patients with patellar instability, there is often a sensation of patellar slippage or a feeling of actual bony subluxation, particularly with twisting, cutting, or pivoting activity. Only rarely, however, will a runner turn sharply enough to sustain a dynamic force sufficient to cause an acute dislocation of the patella.

PHYSICAL EXAMINATION

The positive findings in PFP are often subtle, and it is not always clear if they correlate with the patients' symptoms. Clinical studies have not been able to consistently demonstrate biomechanical or alignment differences between patients with PFP and healthy individuals.[23–25] Some of this relates to the difficulty defining where the range of normal alignment ends and malalignment begins. Physical examination for static malalignment has a place in clinical and scientific evaluation. However, many of these malalignments change once movement is initiated. Furthermore, additional malalignment may exist during movement as a result of poor muscular control of the segments.[16] Given this, the authors still believe that the physical examination, when systematically performed, can highlight predisposing static and dynamic factors to patellofemoral malalignment that are important to address in the design of an individualized treatment program.[26]

Standing Examination

Static alignment

The anatomic alignment of the pelvis and lower extremity may play a role in the development of PFPS in some individuals, and is referred to as "static alignment" because it is identifiable when the patient is not moving. Static alignment is not easily modified with conservative rehabilitation. Alignment of the lower extremity is evaluated by noting evidence of femoral anteversion; knee position (genu varum, valgum, or recurvatum); external tibial rotation; and foot and ankle weight-bearing alignment. A common clinical measurement of the alignment of the lower extremity is the Q-angle. The Q-angle is formed by the line connecting the anterosuperior iliac spine to the center of the patella and the line connecting the center of the patella to the middle of the anterior tibial tuberosity. This angle is thought to represent the line of action of the quadriceps force. Although many sources report that a Q-angle greater than 16° is a risk factor for developing PFPS, the literature is inconsistent in supporting this finding.[16,24] Although some investigators[27,28] have found a difference between the Q-angles of men and women, a study by Grelsamer and colleagues[29] concluded that when measurement data are corrected for the average height between men and women, the difference in the Q-angle between men and women disappears.

Dynamic alignment

Dynamic malalignment may exist during movement as a result of poor muscular control of the lower extremity segments. Dynamic alignment can be tested by having the runner step slowly upon and down from a 6-inch stool or perform single-leg squats. The presence of any abnormal movements of the patella as it engages and disengages the trochlea, and any body shifting, trunk rotation, or loss of hip control are noted. The "dynamic Q-angle" that causes dysfunction has been described. The concept of poor dynamic alignment took form when clinicians observed a consistent pattern when patients performed a single-leg squat or step-down of excessive contralateral pelvic drop; hip adduction and internal rotation; knee abduction; and tibial external rotation and hyperpronation. Several investigators have described this movement pattern and its link to PFPS.[30–32] Dynamic magnetic resonance imaging (MRI) has shown that during weight bearing, PFPS subjects had greater femoral internal rotation than control subjects.[33]

This concept supports the idea that poor control of the femur may contribute to PFPS symptoms in some patients. The excessive frontal and transverse plane motion seen in women during functional tasks has been attributed to weakness in the hip abductors and external rotators.[30,31,34,35] Gluteus medius weakness allows the contralateral pelvis to drop, and puts the stance leg in an adducted position; this is accompanied by excessive internal rotation of the femur and tibia and hyperpronation of the subtalar joint.[36,37] Normally the patella travels smoothly through the trochlear groove and follows a straight or slightly curved path. An abrupt or sudden lateral movement of the patella as the knee nears full extension is considered abnormal. Called a positive J-sign, this movement is caused by excessive lateral forces as the patella exits the femoral trochlea at 10° to 30° of flexion,[6,38] and is seen in a small number of patients with patellar malalignment and in the majority of patients with frank patellofemoral instability.

Sitting Examination

In the sitting position, patellar height for signs of alta or baja position can also be assessed. A prominent infrapatellar fat pad often accompanies patella alta, as does genu recurvatum. Patella alta is more frequently seen in women and is a common finding in a congenitally subluxing patella, as it causes the patella to enter the femoral sulcus late in knee flexion. Patella baja is rarer and is sometimes seen as a complication of anterior cruciate ligament reconstruction. The path of the patellar tendon insertion into the tibial tuberosity is also noted. When the tibial tubercle is situated more laterally than normal, such that the patellar tendon descends at an angle rather than directly downward, proximal external tibial torsion is present.

Dynamic patellar tracking is a measure of patellar instability. During this evaluation, the examiner asks the seated patient to actively extend the knee from 90° to full extension, and observes the movement pattern of the patella from the front. In most individuals, the patella seems to move straight proximally, with a slight lateral shift near terminal extension (J-sign). The term J-sign describes the path of the patella with mal-tracking. Instead of moving superiorly with knee extension, the patella suddenly deviates laterally at terminal extension as it exits the trochlear groove, to create an inverted J-shaped path.[22,39]

Supine Examination

Leg length discrepancies can be screened by measuring the distance from the anterior superior iliac spine to the highest point of the medial malleolus. Leg length discrepancy greater than 1.0 cm may have adverse effects on the lower extremity while running.[40] The knee joint is then observed and palpated for any swelling. As little as 20 to 30 mL of fluid in the knee joint can inhibit VMO function.[41] It is unusual, however, to have any more than a mild synovitis of the knee with chronic extensor mechanism problems.

The examination then focuses on palpation of the patella and peripatellar soft tissues for tenderness. The lateral retinaculum interdigitates with fibers from the vastus lateralis and ITB, and tenderness is frequently palpated in this area related to the chronic, recurrent stress of a maligned patella.[38,42] Several studies have presented evidence of nerve damage and hyperinnervation into the lateral retinaculum in patients with patellofemoral malalignment.[43,44] In these individuals, the neural growth factor is overexpressed in the nerve fiber and vessel wall, and stimulates the release of substance P in the free nerve endings.[44] This condition is often associated with tenderness along the medial patellar facet, and less often, the lateral patellar facet. These areas are best palpated by curling the fingers around the border of the patella. The examiner next palpates along the patellar tendon, specifically at its attachment to the distal pole of the patella. Patellar tendinitis is demonstrated by tenderness to palpation in this area. Tenderness directly ventral or dorsal to the patellar tendon is associated with patellar bursitis and tendinopathy, whereas tenderness along either side of the patellar tendon is associated with inflammation of the fat pad of Hoffa. Less commonly, tenderness is located at the proximal pole of the patella at the quadriceps insertion, indicating quadriceps tendinitis.

Close observation of the patella in relation to the femur is continued. Grelsamer and McConnell[10] describe 4 components that are believed to affect patellar position statically or dynamically: glide, tilt, rotation, and anterior-posterior position. The glide test is an assessment of lateral/medial displacement of the patella, and measures the distance from the midpole of the patella to the medial and lateral femoral epicondyles with the knee flexed to 20°. The patella may sit equidistant to the condyles, but moves laterally when the quadriceps contract, indicating a dynamic problem. The glide component is examined by use of a tape measure to record the distance from the midpatella to the lateral femoral epicondyle and the distance from the midpatella to the medial femoral epicondyle. The midpatella point is determined by visual assessment.[10] A 5-mm lateral displacement of the patella caused a 50% decrease in vastus medialis oblique tension.[45] While it is common for patients with PFP to have some degree of lateral displacement, these clinical measurements should be interpreted with caution, because they may not be a true reflection of anatomic position. Powers and colleagues[46] found that the clinical assessment of patellar glide (medial/lateral displacement) overestimated the true amount of lateral displacement assessed on MRI.

Patellar tilt compares the height of the anterior aspect of the medial patellar border with the height of the anterior aspect of the lateral patellar border. This tilt is considered normal when the 2 borders are level in the frontal plane. In mild tilt, more than 50% of the depth of the lateral border can be palpated but the posterior surface is not palpable; and in more severe tilt less than 50% of the depth of the lateral border can be palpated. To determine the presence of a dynamic tilt problem, an active contraction is simulated by passively moving the patella medially. If the depth of the lateral border becomes more difficult to palpate, a dynamic tilt is present. If the lateral tilt is severe, this can lead to lateral patellar compression syndrome, sometimes requiring surgical release (**Fig. 1**).

Rotational measurements help to determine any deviation of the long axis of the patella from the long axis of the femur, and are believed to be another indication that a particular part of the retinaculum is tight and a potential source of symptoms.

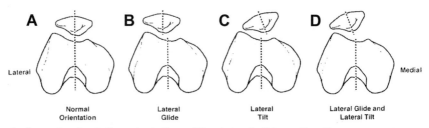

Fig. 1. Example of patellar orientation with a lateral glide and/or tilt component.

In normal rotation a line connecting the superior and inferior poles of the patella is parallel to the long axis of the femur. If the inferior pole is medial to the long axis of the femur, this signifies internal rotation; if the inferior pole of the patella is lateral to the long axis of the femur, this signifies external rotation.

The evaluation of anteroposterior (A-P) alignment is to assess if the inferior pole is tilted posteriorly compared with the superior pole. Such tilting can irritate the fat pad and is common in patients who have pain on extension or hyperextension of the knee, because the inferior pole gets buried in the fat pad. These patients are often diagnosed as having a patellar tendonitis, and usually have pain with quad sets and straight leg raises. A-P tilt occurs when the distal one-third of the patella, or the inferior pole of the patella, is not as clear to palpate as the superior one-third and superior pole. These individuals often present with a dimple in their knees. Dynamically anterior-posterior tilt can be determined during a maximal quadriceps contraction. If the inferior pole disappears as a dimple, then the test is positive.

Also important is assessment of patellar mobility.[47] The test is performed with the knee flexed 20° to 30° and the quadriceps relaxed. The test can be done either by resting the patient's knee over the examiner's thigh or with a small pillow underneath the patient's knee. The patella is divided into 4 longitudinal quadrants, and the patella is displaced medially and laterally with the examiner's thumb and index finger to determine the amount of patellar tightness (**Fig. 2**). A lateral displacement of 3 quadrants suggests an incompetent medial restraint. A lateral displacement of 4 quadrants defines a dislocatable patella. A medial displacement of only 1 quadrant indicates a tight lateral retinaculum and usually correlates with an abnormal passive patellar tilt test. There is an association between patellar hypomobility and a tight ITB.[48] Medial displacement of 3 or 4 quadrants suggests a more globally hypermobile patella without tightness of the lateral restraints, and is often seen in patients with other stigmata of generalized ligamentous laxity. Hypermobility with lateral patellar glide is correlated with laxity of the medial patellofemoral ligament or patellomeniscal ligament, and is often noted in association with patellar subluxation. During these maneuvers, the examiner should look not only for patellar mobility but also for any associated apprehension. When positive, this is a very specific test for patellar instability.

The ligamentous stability of both knees is assessed, particularly if there is a previous history of knee injury. Both anterior and posterior cruciate deficiencies are associated with peripatellar pain. Careful evaluation for meniscal pathology is noted by palpation of the medial and lateral joint lines and McMurray testing. Joint-line tenderness can be present with patellar pathology if there is an associated synovitis, and does not necessarily indicate a meniscal injury or femorotibial arthritis.[10] Identification of a symptomatic synovial plica is equally important.

Hip range of motion, femoral acetabular impingement tests, and the Faber maneuver should be thoroughly assessed to rule out referred pain to the knee from

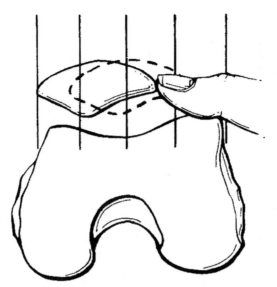

Fig. 2. Assessment of patellar mobility medially and laterally. (*From* Assessment of patellar mobility medially and laterally. In: DeLee JC, Drez D, editors. Orthopaedic sports medicine, vol. 2. Philadelphia (PA): W.B. Saunders Co; 1994. p. 1179; with permission.)

intra-articular hip pathology. Internal rotation that exceeds external rotation is suggestive of femoral anteversion, and following this, soft tissue length should be measured in the hamstrings and hip flexors.

Side-Lying Examination

In the side-lying position, with the knee flexed at 20°, the lateral retinaculum can be evaluated for excessive tightness by passively moving the patella in a medial direction.[10] The superficial retinacular fibers are believed to be tight if the femoral condyle is not easily exposed. To test the deep fibers, the hand is placed on the middle of the patella, the slack of any lateral glide is removed, and an anteroposterior pressure on the medial border of the patella is applied. The lateral border of the patella should move freely away from the femur, and on palpation the tension in the retinacular fibers should be similar.

In this position ITB tightness can be evaluated with Ober's test, and the gluteus medius can be tested for strength deficits.

Prone Examination

This position allows a more accurate assessment of rearfoot and forefoot alignment, subtalar position, gastroc-soleus, and quadriceps muscle length.

Observational Gait Analysis

Observational gait analysis is one of the most important aspects of the examination—the evaluation of dynamic function by observing the runner's angle of gait while walking and running. In more complicated cases, it may be helpful to use treadmill running or even more sophisticated video taping to analyze the runner's gait. The findings of Thijs and colleagues[49] suggest that an excessive impact-shock during heel-strike and at the propulsion phase of running may contribute to an increased risk of developing PFP. Dierks and colleagues[50] have also shown that runners with PFPS displayed weaker hip abductor muscles that were associated with an increase in hip adduction during running. This relationship became more pronounced at the end of the run.

DIAGNOSTIC STUDIES

The diagnosis of PFPS depends primarily on the history of the patient. Radiography is an adjunct to history and physical examination. It is important to obtain radiographs in the runner who has apparent PFP and does not demonstrate improvement after several weeks of conservative treatment, or if there has been a history of recent trauma or dislocation. Radiographic findings do not correlate well with clinical complaints and frequently the injured side is difficult to differentiate from the uninjured side.[51] When imaging is indicated, plain films of the knee (weight-bearing A-P, weight-bearing lateral, and axial view) are useful to rule out other sources of anterior knee pain, including bipartite patella, osteoarthritis, loose bodies, and occult fractures.

On standard A-P radiographs of the knee, one can identify accessory ossification centers, degenerative joint disease, and other unrelated conditions, such as bone tumors.[52]

The lateral view is most helpful for assessing patellar height. There is a plethora of measurement techniques described in the literature for this purpose.[10] The Blackburne and Peel[53] technique is easy to use and fairly reliable. This technique measures the distance from the tibial plateau to the inferior pole, which should equal the length of the patellar articular surface (**Fig. 3**). Normal values are approximately 1.0, with higher values indicating patellar alta. The technique should be used with caution in adolescent patients with skeletally immature proximal tibial epiphysis, certain patellar morphotypes with short articular surface, or when there is an abnormal slope of the tibial plateau.[10]

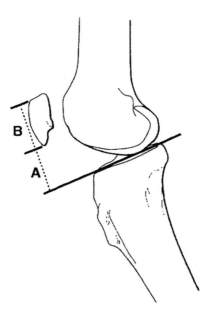

Fig. 3. Technique of Blackburn and Peel to assess patella alta on lateral radiographs of the knee.

Axial or Merchant views of the patellofemoral joint are recommended with the knee flexed 30°.[10] Some subluxation can be detected at 30° that could be missed at 45°. This view allows evaluation of degenerative changes in the patellofemoral joint, osteo-chondritis dissecans of the patella, patellar morphology, dysplasia of the trochlear groove, and accessory ossification centers and ectopic calcifications in the retinac-ulum. The position and orientation of the patella relative to the trochlear groove are also evaluated with the sulcus angle, congruence angle, and the patellar tilt angle.

The sulcus angle measures the angle of the bony trochlea. With the knee flexed at 30° to 45°, the normal sulcus angle is approximately 140°.[54] Patellar instability is asso-ciated with a more shallow trochlea, whereas too steep a trochlea is associated with patellar pain without instability.[55]

The congruence angle is an index of medial/lateral subluxation of the patella within the trochlear groove, similar to the physical examination assessment of patellar glide, and in nondislocators the average angle is −6° (standard deviation 11°) (**Fig. 4**A).[42] Although this measurement has been widely used, drawing and bisecting an angle can prove to be time-consuming and difficult with both plain radiographs and digital radiography. A new axial linear displacement measurement presented in the study by Urch and colleagues[56] provides a simple alternative method for evaluating the posi-tion of the patella relative to the trochlear groove that is similar to that of the congru-ence angle measurement (see **Fig. 4**B).

The patellar tilt angle is an index of the medial/lateral tilt of the plane of the patella relative to the femur (**Fig. 5**). In the normal patellofemoral joint, the angle formed by the lateral patellar facet and any horizontal line should open laterally, whereas in patients with patellar subluxation the lines used to define the angle are parallel or open medi-ally.[57] For this evaluation to be accurate and repeatable, the radiograph must be taken with the foot vertical and the cassette maintained parallel to the ground. If the patient exhibits external tibial torsion, the natural position of the feet is maintained. A tilt angle between 0° and 5° is normal, 5° to 10° is borderline, and an angle greater than 10° is considered abnormal. In a study by Grelsamer and colleagues[58] abnormal tilt was detected in 85% of patients suffering from malalignment pain. The 15% of patients whose malalignment was not detected exhibited either abnormal tilt that became normal at 30° of flexion or malalignment that was not related to tilt (ie, patella alta or lateral displacement).

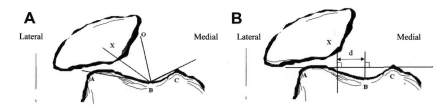

Fig. 4. (*A*) Congruence angle. Line BO is the bisector of angle ABC. Line BX passes through the lowest point on the median ridge of the patella. Angle OBX is the congruence angle. If line BX falls to the medial side of line BO, the angle is expressed as negative degrees. If it falls to the lateral side of line BO, it is expressed as positive degrees. (*B*) A reference line is drawn by connecting the most anterior aspects of the lateral (A) and medial (C) trochlear facets. A line is drawn perpendicularly from the depth of the sulcus (B) through the refer-ence line (AC). Another line is drawn perpendicularly from the posterior aspect of the patellar spine (X) through the reference line. To obtain the lateral displacement measure-ment, the distance (d) between the 2 intersections is measured.

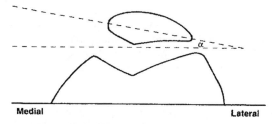

Medial   Lateral

Fig. 5. Patellar tilt angle. The tilt angle is measured by a line joining the corners of the patella and any horizontal line. (*From* Grelsamer RP, McConnell J. The patella. Gaithersburg (MD): Aspen Publishers; 1998. *Adapted from* Grelsamer, RP, Bazos AN, Proctor CS. Radiographic analysis of patellar tilt. J Bone Joint Surg Br. 1993 Sep ;75(5):822–4; with permission.)

Because the patella usually becomes unstable as it nears extension, a lateralized patella may not be detected by an axial-view radiograph that requires the knee be flexed to at least 30°. Thus if surgery is contemplated and plain films are negative, an MRI scan or computed tomography (CT) scan should be used to further evaluate patellar tracking. Serial CT scans taken at knee flexion angles in the range of 0° to 30° can provide even greater information about the tracking of the patella in the trochlear groove. Measurements of sulcus angle, congruence angle, and patellar tilt angle can be performed on CT scans just as they can be performed on conventional axial radiographs, and may be helpful in understanding the patient with a difficult patellofemoral problem.[59,60] Three patterns of malalignment can be characterized by the congruence angle and patellar tilt angle: lateral subluxation without lateral tilt, subluxation with tilt, and tilt without subluxation.

Kinematic studies can also be accomplished with MRI[61,62] without exposure to radiation. In addition to defining tracking abnormalities, MRI is particularly helpful in assessing any degenerative joint changes, such as cartilage fissuring or thinning, subchondral bone marrow edema, subchondral cysts, and other pathologic entities such as synovial plica and patellar tendinitis. A new method using real-time MRI allows measurement of patellofemoral joint motion during weight-bearing and non–weight-bearing dynamic tasks (**Fig. 6**).[63] The aim is to define the cause of PFP using real-time MRI in experimental research. Single-slice, spiral, real-time MR images of all subjects performing knee flexion/extension were obtained in a 0.5-T open MRI scanner (**Fig. 7**).

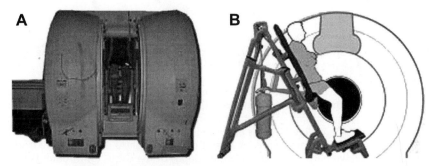

Fig. 6. (*A*) Open-bore MRI scanner with subject performing a weight-bearing squat. (*B*) Side view of scanner and backrest used to stabilize subjects as they moved in the scanner. Subjects supported about 90% of their body weight.

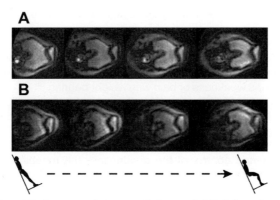

Fig. 7. (*A*) Real-time MR images of the patellofemoral (PF) joint of a pain-free control subject during upright, weight-bearing knee extension. (*B*) Real-time MR images of the PF joint of a subject with pain during upright, weight-bearing knee extension. Notice the lateral position and rotation of the patella relative to the femur.

REHABILITATION

The management of PFPS should include a comprehensive rehabilitation program. Symptom control (activity modification, nonsteroidal anti-inflammatory drugs, ice or cold application, patellar taping, or patellar bracing) is the first stage, then patients should be classified by suspected contributing mechanisms: abnormal patellofemoral joint mechanics, altered lower extremity alignment and/or motion, and overuse.[7]

Abnormal Patellofemoral Tracking and Alignment

Tightness of soft tissue structures
Soft tissue inflexibilities, particularly in the hamstrings and ITB, can also affect normal patella excursion and should be addressed.[7,64] Soft tissue mobilization and stretching techniques are also important to address tight retinaculum structures contributing to abnormal patellar tracking.

Decreased patellar mobility
Patellar mobilization techniques should be performed if evidence of decreased patellar mobility is noted. These techniques should be performed with care to prevent excessive patellofemoral joint compression.

Quadriceps muscle strengthening
Restoration of quadriceps strength and function has been demonstrated to be a significant contributing factor to recovery from patellofemoral symptoms.[65] However, the mechanism by which strengthening improves PFP symptoms and functional ability is not entirely clear.

Choosing the correct exercises to prescribe for an individual with PFP requires an understanding of patellofemoral joint biomechanics. During open chain exercises, the amount of quadriceps muscle force required to extend the knee steadily increases as the knee moves from 90° to full knee extension.[11] In addition, the patellofemoral joint contact area decreases as the knee extends, thereby increasing patellofemoral joint stress. By contrast, during closed chain exercises the quadriceps muscle force is minimal at full knee extension and therefore, patellofemoral joint stresses are reduced.[11] Examples of closed chain exercises include lunges, wall slides, and leg press machines.

Both open and closed chain strengthening exercises should be performed so that strengthening can be performed throughout a large arc of motion. Isometrics and open kinetic chain exercises, such as knee extensions, are recommended if there is significant quadriceps weakness or pain with weight bearing.[66] As quickly as possible, however, patients should be progressed to the core of the rehabilitation program that includes a closed kinetic chain quadriceps strengthening regimen, which is more effective than isokinetic joint isolation and open chain exercises in improving function.[67,68]

To improve eccentric control of the quadriceps, the rehabilitation program also should include exercises performed while standing on one leg. In this position, the lower abdominals and the gluteals work together to maintain a level pelvis, simulating the activity of the stance phase of gait.[10] Activation of the lower abdominal and oblique muscles helps to decrease the anterior rotation of the pelvis and the resultant internal rotation of the femur (step-down exercises: **Fig. 8**).

In addition, Souza and Powers[69] have demonstrated abnormal hip kinematics in women with PFP that seem to be the result of diminished hip-muscle performance rather than altered femoral structure. The results suggest that assessment of

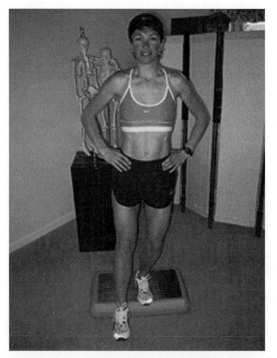

Fig. 8. Step-down exercise. The pelvis should remain parallel with the floor; the hip, knee and foot should be aligned, avoiding excessive hip adduction or internal rotation. The goal is to activate the gluteal and quadricep muscles by maintaining erect posture, and avoiding forward body lean as one steps down. Start on a step only a few inches off the ground and increase the distance as stability improves.

hip-muscle performance should be considered in the evaluation and treatment of patellofemoral joint dysfunction.

Role of the Vastus Medialis Obliquus

Isolated recruitment of the VMO, proposed by many therapists, has not been proven to occur with exercises that are commonly prescribed for the treatment of PFP. One electromyographic study examined 9 commonly used strengthening exercises and found that the activity of the VMO was not significantly greater than that of the vastus lateralis, the vastus intermedius, and the vastus medialis longus, suggesting that isolated recruitment or strengthening of the VMO through selected exercises is unrealistic and probably translates into a general quadriceps muscle strengthening effect.[7,70]

Patellar Taping

Correcting abnormal patella posture using the Grelsamer and McConnell[10] taping technique is one way of optimizing the entry of the patella into the trochlea, and is a transitional step in the rehabilitation process in those patients who are unable to perform strengthening exercises due to their pain. Taping the patella of symptomatic individuals during stair ascent and descent exercises can diminish symptoms by 50%. In addition, it has been shown to increase quadriceps activity and permit increased loading of the knee joint.[11]

Patellar Braces

Patients with patellar pain may report decreased pain from wearing properly fitted dynamic patellar stabilization braces. Powers and colleagues[71] found that 50% of subjects experienced an improvement in symptoms with the use of patellar stabilizing braces. Further study[64] evaluating the same brace, however, did not find it was able to consistently correct patellar tracking patterns as measured quantitatively by kinematic MRI. However, a more recent study by Draper and colleagues[63] evaluated women with PFP during dynamic, weight-bearing knee extension, and assessed the effects of knee braces on patellofemoral motion with real-time magnetic resonance images of the patellofemoral joints of 36 women volunteers. The results suggest that different subsets of women with PFP exist and that bracing seems to have a mechanical effect in only one group compared with the controls: those with abnormal kinematics. With application of the brace, the lateral translation and tilt of the patella were reduced but were not restored to normal. A simple patellar sleeve provided more mild correction of lateral translation of the patella but did not alter patellar tilt.

Lower Kinetic Chain Problems

Subtalar joint pronation

Excessive pronation whether secondary to abnormal compensation as a result of abnormal structure in the trunk or lower extremity, or secondary to pathology in the foot itself, should also be addressed. Excessive pronation can increase the Q-angle, causing a dynamic abduction moment at the knee and a consequent increase in the laterally directed force on the patella. It should be noted that not all patients with excessive pronation need an orthotic. In fact, a recent study[72] showed that although foot orthoses are superior to flat inserts according to participants' overall perception, they are similar to physiotherapy and do not improve outcomes when added to physiotherapy in the short-term management of PFP.

In those runners who seem to benefit from an orthotic, a custom-molded orthotic for maximal biomechanical control is recommended. Most over-the-counter orthotic devices have been designed to address primary control of rearfoot motion.

Three-dimensional studies, however, have shown that forefoot stability may play an integral role in rearfoot stability.[73] These studies indicate that instability in the forefoot at push-off may create instability in the rearfoot. For this reason an orthotic that extends all the way to the sulcus or web-space of the toes is considered crucial for control of forefoot instability in runners.[10]

Hip internal rotation

The functional significance of an internally rotated femur is that the trochlear groove can rotate beneath the patella, placing the patella in a fairly lateral position. If it is observed that the femur collapses into internal rotation during gait, and this motion seems to originate from the pelvis, then strengthening of the external rotators including gluteus maximus, gluteus medius, and the deep rotators may be indicated. If the femur remains in a constant state of internal rotation during the gait cycle (rather than collapsing inward), femoral anteversion should be suspected. As femoral anteversion is a fixed bony deformity, little can be done from a nonsurgical standpoint to correct this abnormality.

Gait Deviations

The restoration of normal gait function is essential to the overall treatment plan. Preliminary work from Noehren and Davis[74] suggests that gait retraining with real-time visual feedback can alter faulty mechanics, such as increased hip adduction and internal rotation and pelvic drop. Research in cadavers has shown that decreasing hip adduction or internal rotation decreases the compression on the lateral facet of the patella.[75,76] In addition, decreased pelvic drop reduces the strain on the ITB, which in turn reduces its lateral force on the patella and allows more normal alignment.[77]

Overuse

The lack of significant findings on physical examination (ie, normal patellar mechanics, normal lower extremity function) suggests that the source of PFP symptoms may be related to overuse. This overuse is often seen in an athletic population. The treatment program should focus on relative rest with activity modification. The training program also should be evaluated for obvious errors, including increasing exercise intensity too quickly, inadequate time for recovery, and excessive hill work.

Most runners with PFP and malalignment, including those with minor instability problems, will respond to nonoperative treatment. The lateral retinacular release is perhaps the most frequently performed surgical procedure, but is only indicated if a major contributor to malalignment is a tight lateral retinaculum causing isolated patellar tilt.[47] A common complication of lateral retinacular release is an incomplete release, which most commonly is the failure to release the patellar tibial portion of the lateral retinaculum along with the patellofemoral portion. By contrast, an over-zealous release can lead to medial subluxation or dislocation. A lateral release will not correct more global patellar hypermobility or an abnormal anatomic Q-angle. In these cases, more extensive realignment surgery may be contemplated but is unlikely to permit a return to serious running.[14,42]

REFERENCES

1. Van Mechelen W. Running injuries: a review of the epidemiologic literature. Sports Med 1992;14(5):320–35.
2. Taunton JE, Ryan MB, Clement DB, et al. A retrospective case-control analysis of 2002 running injuries. Br J Sports Med 2002;36:95.

3. Holmes WS, Clancy WG. Clinical classification of patellofemoral pain and dysfunction. J Orthop Sports Phys Ther 1998;28:299–306.

4. Goodfellow J, Hungerford DS, Zindel M. Patellofemoral joint mechanics and pathology. 1. Functional anatomy of the patellofemoral joint. J Bone Joint Surg Br 1976;58:287–90.

5. Walsh WM. Patellofemoral joint. In: DeLee JC, Drez D, editors. Orthopaedic sports medicine, vol. 2. Philadelphia: W.B. Saunders Co; 1994. p. 1163–248.

6. Hughston JC, Walsh WM, Puddu G. Patellar subluxation and dislocation. Philadelphia: W.B. Saunders; 1984.

7. Fredericson M, Powers CM. Practical management of patellofemoral pain. Clin J Sport Med 2002;12:36–8.

8. Powers C, Maffucci R, Hampton S. Rearfoot posture in subjects with patellofemoral pain. J Orthop Sports Phys Ther 1995;22:155–60.

9. Bose K, Kanagasuntherum R, Osman M. Vastus medialis oblique: an anatomical and physiologic study. Orthopedics 1980;3:880–3.

10. Grelsamer RP, McConnell J. The patella. Gaithersburg (MD): Aspen Publishers; 1998.

11. Powers CM. Rehabilitation of patellofemoral joint disorders: a critical review. J Orthop Sports Phys Ther 1998;28(5):3453–4.

12. Van Tiggelen D, Cowan S, Coorevits P, et al. Delayed vastus medialis obliquus to vastus lateralis onset timing contributes to the development of patellofemoral pain in previously healthy men: a prospective study. Am J Sports Med 2009; 37(6):1099–105.

13. Sanchis-Alfonso V, Rosello-Sastre E, Martinez-Sanjuan V. Pathogenesis of anterior knee pain syndrome and functional patellofemoral instability in the active young. Am J Knee Surg 1999;12:29–40.

14. James SL, Jones DC. Biomechanical aspects of distance running injuries. In: Cavanagh PR, editor. Biomechanics of distance running. Champaign (IL): Human Kinetics Books; 1990. p. 249–69.

15. Root M, Orien W, Weed J. Clinical biomechanics, vol. 11. Los Angeles (CA): Clinical Biomechanics Corp; 1977.

16. Earl JE, Vetter CS. Patellofemoral pain. Phys Med Rehabil Clin N Am 2007;18: 439–58.

17. Besier TF, Gold GE, Delp SL, et al. The influence of femoral internal and external rotation on cartilage stresses within the patellofemoral joint. J Orthop Res 2008; 26(12):1627–35.

18. Heino Brechter J, Powers CM. Patellofemoral stress during walking in persons with and without patellofemoral pain. Med Sci Sports Exerc 2002;34:1582–93.

19. Fredericson M. Patellofemoral pain syndrome. In: O'Connor F, Wilder R, editors. The textbook of running medicine. New York: The McGraw Hill Companies; 2001. p. 169–80.

20. Brushøj C, Hölmich P, Nielsen MB, et al. Acute patellofemoral pain: aggravating activities, clinical examination, MRI and ultrasound findings. Br J Sports Med 2008;42(1):64–7.

21. Dye SF. The pathophysiology of patellofemoral pain: a tissue homeostasis perspective. Clin Orthop Relat Res 2005;436:100–10.

22. Post WR. Clinical evaluation of patients with patellofemoral disorders. Arthroscopy 1999;15(8):841–51.

23. Kannus P, Nittymaki S. Which factors predict outcome in the nonoperative treatment of patellofemoral pain syndrome? A prospective follow-up study. Med Sci Sports Exerc 1994;26(3):289–96.

24. Messier SP, Davis SE, Curl WW, et al. Etiologic factors associated with patellofemoral pain in runners. Med Sci Sports Exerc 1991;23(9):1008–15.

25. Thomee R, Renstrom P, Karlsson J, et al. Patellofemoral pain syndrome in young women. I. A clinical analysis of alignment, pain, parameters, common symptoms and functional activity level. Scand J Med Sci Sports 1995;5(4):237–44.

26. Fredericson M, Yoon K. Physical examination and patellofemoral pain syndrome. Am J Phys Med Rehabil 2006;85(3):234–43.

27. Hvid I, Andersen LI. The quadriceps angle and its relation to femoral torsion. Acta Orthop Scand 1982;53:577–9.

28. Livingston LA. The quadriceps angle: a review of the literature. J Orthop Sports Phys Ther 1998;28:105–9.

29. Grelsamer RP, Dubey A, Weinstein CH. Men and women have similar Q-angles: a clinical and trigonometric evaluation. J Bone Joint Surg Br 2005;87:1498–501.

30. Ireland M, Willson J, Ballantyne B, et al. Hip strength in females with and without patellofemoral pain. J Orthop Sports Phys Ther 2003;33:671–6.

31. Powers C. The influence of altered lower-extremity kinematics on patellofemoral joint dysfunction: a theoretical perspective. J Orthop Sports Phys Ther 2003;33:639–46.

32. Riegger-Krugh C, Keysor J. Skeletal malalignments of the lower quarter: correlated and compensatory motions and postures. J Orthop Sports Phys Ther 1996;2:164–70.

33. Powers C, Ward S, Frederiscon M, et al. Patellofemoral kinematics during weight-bearing and non-weight bearing knee extension in persons with lateral subluxation of the patella: a preliminary study. J Orthop Sports Phys Ther 2003;33(11):677–85.

34. Zeller B, McCrory J, Kibler B, et al. Differences in kinematics and electromyographic activity between men and women during the single-legged squat. Am J Sports Med 2003;31:449–56.

35. Leetun D, Ireland M, Willson J, et al. Core stability measures as risk factors for lower extremity in athletes. Med Sci Sports Exerc 2004;36:926–34.

36. Host J, Craig R, Lehman R. Patellofemoral dysfunction in tennis players: a dynamic problem. Clin Sports Med 1995;14:177–203.

37. Sahrmann S. Muscle imbalances in the female athlete. In: Pearl A, editor. The athletic female. Champaign (IL): Human Kinetics; 1993. p. 209–19.

38. Fulkerson JP, Kalenak A, Rosenberg TD, et al. Patellofemoral pain. Instructional Course Outlines. American Academy of Orthopaedic Surgeons; 1994. p. 57–71, Chapter 6.

39. Nissen CW, Cullen MC, Hewett TE, et al. Physical and arthroscopic examination techniques of the patellofemoral joint. J Orthop Sports Phys Ther 1998;28:277–85.

40. McCaw ST. Leg length inequality. Implications for running injury prevention. Sports Med 1992;14(6):422–9.

41. de Andrade JR, Grant C, Dixon AS. Joint distention and reflex muscle inhibition in the knee. J Bone Joint Surg Am 1965;47:313–22.

42. Merchant AC. Patellofemoral malalignment and instabilities. In: Ewing JW, editor. Articular cartilage and knee joint function: basic science and arthroscopy. New York: Raven Press Ltd; 1990. p. 79–91.

43. Mori Y, Fujimoto A, Okumo H, et al. Lateral retinaculum release in adolescent patellofemoral disorders: its relationship to peripheral nerve injury in the lateral retinaculum. Bull Hosp Jt Dis Orthop Inst 1991;51:218–29.

44. Sanchis-Alfonso V, Roselló-Sastre E, Revert F. Neural growth factor expression in the lateral retinaculum in painful patellofemoral malalignment. Acta Orthop Scand 2001;72:146–9.

45. Ahmed A, Shi S, Hyder A, et al. The effect of quadriceps tension characteristics on the patellar tracking pattern. Trans Annu Meet Orthop Res Soc [Atlanta (GA)] 1988;13:280.

46. Powers CM, Mortenson S, Nishimoto D, et al. Criterion-related validity of a clinical measurement to determine the medial/lateral component of patellar orientation. J Orthop Sports Phys Ther 1999;29(7):372–7.

47. Kolowich PA, Paulos LE, Rosenberg TD, et al. Lateral release of the patella: indications and contraindications. Am J Sports Med 1990;18:359–65.

48. Puniello MS. Iliotibial band tightness and medial patellar glide in patients with patellofemoral dysfunction. J Orthop Sports Phys Ther 1993;17:144–8.

49. Thijs Y, De Clercq D, Roosen P, et al. Gait-related intrinsic risk factors for patellofemoral pain in novice recreational runners. Br J Sports Med 2008;42(6):466–71.

50. Dierks TA, Manal KT, Hamill J, et al. Proximal and distal influences on hip and knee kinematics in runners with patellofemoral pain during a prolonged run. J Orthop Sports Phys Ther 2008;38(8):448–56.

51. Haim A, Yaniv M, Dekel S, et al. Patellofemoral pain syndrome: validity of clinical and radiological features. Clin Orthop Relat Res 2006;451:223–8.

52. Bergman AG, Fredericson M. MR imaging of stress reactions, muscle injuries, and other overuse injuries in runners. Magn Reson Imaging Clin N Am 1999; 7(1):151–73.

53. Blackburne JS, Peel TE. A new method of measuring patellar height. J Bone Joint Surg Br 1977;59:241–2.

54. Brattström H. The picture of the femoro-patellar joint in recurrent dislocation of the patella. Acta Orthop Scand 1963;33:373–5.

55. Buard J, Benoit J, Lortat-Jacob A, et al. Les trochlées fémorales creuses [Dysplastic trochlea]. Rev Chir Orthop 1981;67:721–9 [in French].

56. Urch SE, Tritle BA, Shelbourne KD, et al. Axial linear patellar displacement: a new measurement of patellofemoral congruence. Am J Sports Med 2009;37(5):970–3.

57. Laurin CA, Levesque HP, Dussault R, et al. The abnormal lateral patellofemoral angle. J Bone Joint Surg Am 1978;60:55–60.

58. Grelsamer RP, Bazos AN, Proctor CS. A roentgenographic analysis of patellar tilt. J Bone Joint Surg Br 1993;75:822–4.

59. Schutzer SF, Rasby GR, Fulkerson JP. Computed tomographic classification of patellofemoral pain patients. Orthop Clin North Am 1986;17:235–48.

60. Płomiński J, Zabicka M, Kwiatkowski K. Functional evaluation of patello-femoral incongruence by computer tomography. Ortop Traumatol Rehabil 2004;6(3): 323–30.

61. Brossman J, Muhle C, Schroder C, et al. Motion-triggered MR imaging: evaluation of patellar tracking patterns during active and passive knee extension. Radiology 1993;187:205–12.

62. Shellock FG, Stone KR, Crues JV. Development and clinical application of kinematic MRI of the patellofemoral joint using an extremity MR system. Med Sci Sports Exerc 1999;31(5):788–91.

63. Draper CE, Besier TF, Santos JM, et al. Using real-time MRI to quantify altered joint kinematics in subjects with patellofemoral pain and to evaluate the effects of a patellar brace or sleeve on joint motion. J Orthop Res 2009;27(5):571–7.

64. Doucette SA, Goble EM. The effect of exercise on patellar tracking in lateral patellar compression syndrome. Am J Sports Med 1992;20(4):434–40.

65. Natri A, Kannus P, Jarvinen M. Which factors predict the long-term outcome in chronic patellofemoral pain syndrome? A 7-yr prospective follow-up study. Med Sci Sports Exerc 1998;30:1572–7.

66. Escamilla RF, Fleisig GS, Zheng N, et al. Biomechanics of the knee during closed kinetic chain and open kinetic chain exercises. Med Sci Sports Exerc 1998;30(4): 556–9.
67. Doucette SA, Child DD. The effect of open and closed chain exercise and knee joint position on patellar tracking in lateral patellar compression syndrome. J Orthop Sports Phys Ther 1996;23(2):104–10.
68. Steine HA, Brosky T, Reinking MF, et al. A comparison of closed kinetic chain and isokinetic isolation exercise in patients with patellofemoral dysfunction. J Orthop Sports Phys Ther 1996;24(3):136–41.
69. Souza RB, Powers CM. Predictors of hip internal rotation during running: an evaluation of hip strength and femoral structure in women with and without patellofemoral pain. Am J Sports Med 2009;37(3):579–87.
70. Mirzabeigi E, Jordan C, Gronley JK. Isolation of the vastus medialis oblique muscle during exercise. Am J Sports Med 1999;27(1):50–3.
71. Powers CM, Shellock FG, Beering TV. Effect of bracing on patellar kinematics in patients with patellofemoral joint pain. Med Sci Sports Exerc 1999;31(12): 1714–20.
72. Collins N, Crossley K, Beller E, et al. Foot orthoses and physiotherapy in the treatment of patellofemoral pain syndrome: randomized clinical trial. Br J Sports Med 2009;43(3):163–8.
73. Engsberg JR, Andrews JG. Kinematic analysis of the talocalcaneal/talocrural joint during running support. Med Sci Sports Exerc 1987;19:275–83.
74. Noehren B, Davis I, University of Delaware. The effect of gait retraining on hip mechanics, pain and function in runners with patellofemoral pain syndrome, PFPS Retreat. Baltimore (MD); 2009.
75. Huberti HH, Hayes WC. Patellofemoral contact pressures. The influence of q-angle and tendofemoral contact. J Bone Joint Surg Am 1984;66(5):715–24.
76. Lee TQ, Yang BY, Sandusky MD, et al. The effects of tibial rotation on the patellofemoral joint: assessment of the changes in in situ strain in the peripatellar retinaculum and the patellofemoral contact pressures and areas. J Rehabil Res Dev 2001;38(5):463–9.
77. Hamilla J, Millera R, Noehren B, et al. A prospective study of iliotibial band strain in runners. Clin Biomech 2008;23:1018–25.

Stress Fractures in Runners

Mark A. Harrast, MD[a,b,*], Daniel Colonno, MD[c]

KEYWORDS

- Stress fracture • Running injuries
- Overuse injuries • Lower limb

Running has many beneficial effects, including cardiovascular and skeletal health. Poor training technique and a variety of risk factors may predispose runners to lower-limb overuse injuries affecting muscle, tendon, and bone. Injuries to the bone include stress reactions to full-fledged stress fractures. This article is designed to provide an understanding of the general concepts involving bone strain, bone injury risk factor assessment, and evaluation and treatment strategies for the runner with a stress fracture. The second half of the article presents more detail regarding each specific fracture location, grouped as high risk and low risk, common to runners.

PATHOPHYSIOLOGY OF STRESS FRACTURES

An understanding of stress fractures requires an understanding of basic bone biology and the general response of bone remodeling to applied stress. There are two subtypes of bone. Cortical (compact) bone is located in the diaphysis of long bones and the shell of square bones (vertebral bodies and tarsals). Cortical bony turnover is much slower and most stress fractures occur in cortical bone. Cancellous (trabecular) bone is located in the metaphysis and epiphysis of long and square bones. More active remodeling occurs in cancellous bone. Bone mineral density (BMD) measurements are taken of cancellous bone (vertebral body and femoral neck) because of the increased rate of turnover; thus changes in BMD are more readily observed. Stress fractures of cancellous bone correlate with low BMD more so than fractures of cortical bone; therefore, any runner with a cancellous bone stress fracture should have a BMD evaluation.[1]

[a] Seattle Marathon, 1530 Westlake Avenue North, Suite 700, Seattle, WA 98019, USA
[b] University of Washington, UW Medicine Sports and Spine, Box #359721, 325 Ninth Avenue, Seattle, WA 98104, USA
[c] Department of Rehabilitation Medicine, University of Washington, Box #356490, 1959 NE Pacific Street, Seattle, WA 98195, USA
* Corresponding author. University of Washington, UW Medicine Sports and Spine, Box #359721, 325 Ninth Avenue, Seattle, WA 98104.
E-mail address: mharrast@uw.edu

Clin Sports Med 29 (2010) 399–416
doi:10.1016/j.csm.2010.03.001
0278-5919/10/$ – see front matter © 2010 Elsevier Inc. All rights reserved.

sportsmed.theclinics.com

The underlying principle of bone's response to stress is Wolff's law, which states that every change in the form and function of bone leads to changes in its internal architecture and its external form. Simplistically stated, bone is an active substance that adapts to the loads it is placed under. The response of bone to repetitive stress is increased osteoclastic activity over osteoblastic new bone formation, which results in a temporary weakening of bone. The eventual adaptive response is periosteal new bone formation to provide reinforcement. However, if physical stress continues, the osteoclastic activity may predominate resulting initially in microfractures (commonly seen as bone marrow edema on MRI, consistent with a stress reaction) and eventually a true cortical break (stress fracture) may result. Thus, there is a continuum of normal bone strain leading to appropriate remodeling, but if strain becomes excessive or adequate rest is not allowed, stress reaction and eventually stress fracture can result.

It is important to delineate the differences between fatigue and insufficiency type stress fractures. Fatigue fractures are the typical overuse stress fractures observed in athletes and military recruits with normal bone density. Fatigue fractures result from an imbalance in the bone's ability to keep up with skeletal repair from excessive bone strain with progressive accumulation of microdamage. An insufficiency fracture is seen in those with low BMD, such as runners with the female athlete triad; metabolic bone disease; or osteoporosis. Insufficiency fractures result from poor bone remodeling (increased resorption and depressed formation) in response to normal strain. Simply stated, fatigue fractures occur in normal bone under excessive or abnormal strain and insufficiency fractures occur in abnormal bone under normal strain.

RISK FACTORS

Defining the causative risk factors for stress fracture is difficult because there are many interrelated variables that make a risk assessment problematic to independently study. Most studies are case series and many pertain to general overuse injuries in runners, which are not necessarily specifically focused on bone injury. However, these risk factors can be subdivided into extrinsic and intrinsic factors.

Extrinsic Factors

Training variables in runners commonly predispose to stress fractures. An increase in frequency, duration, or intensity of runs is often cited as a primary risk factor. Hard or cambered training surfaces are also factors associated with lower-limb overuse injuries.[2] In a small study, Milgrom demonstrated that treadmill running produced significantly less in vivo tibial strain than over-ground running suggesting treadmill runners are at lower risk for tibial stress fractures.[3] Failure to schedule rest days after higher intensity runs can also contribute to overuse injury risk. Periodization of training is an important coaching technique that maximizes performance gains but also decreases injury risk. Periodization in run training generally follows a 3- to 4-week cycle, with 3 weeks of a progressive buildup of intensity, duration, or distance, followed by an off week of less intense training to allow for rest and the subsequent metabolic training adaptations to occur before entering the next buildup period.

Training in shoes older than 6 months is a risk factor for stress fracture,[4] which is likely related to the decrement in shock absorption as a shoe ages. There is data demonstrating that shock-absorbing foot orthoses decrease the risk for stress fracture in military recruits, though this doesn't necessarily translate to the running athlete.[5,6] A general rule of thumb that most coaches and trainers suggest is changing running shoes every 300 to 500 miles logged to limit excessive risk for lower-limb overuse injuries.

Different running athletes tend to suffer from different locations of stress fractures. Sprinters and hurdlers tend to have more foot fractures, whereas distance runners have more pelvic and long bone fractures.[7]

Intrinsic Factors

It is difficult to definitively determine which specific biomechanical factors affect specific injury rates in runners. Bennell and colleagues[7] demonstrated that smaller calf girth and less muscle mass in the lower limb of female runners was associated with stress fractures. This finding may be because there is less muscle mass to absorb energy, which subsequently transmits to bone. Poor muscular endurance is also considered a risk factor. When muscle fatigues it transmits more force to the adjacent bone. In the military, a more narrow tibial width is a risk factor for stress fracture.[8] Women overall have narrow bones compared with men, which may contribute to the higher risk for stress fracture seen in female runners, though this has not been proven.[9]

Kinematic and kinetic biomechanical variables have also been recently studied as potential risk factors for stress fracture. Running with excessive hip adduction and rear-foot eversion are predictors of tibial stress fractures.[10] It is also hypothesized that lower-limb mechanics during initial loading may relate to peak tibial shock (ie, direct forces transmitted through the tibia).[11] Understanding these kinematic and kinetic factors that predispose to stress fracture may lead to runner gait retraining programs to optimize running mechanics to lessen injury risk.

Other intrinsic risk factors for stress fracture development in runners include those related to gender and bone mineral density. Most studies agree that woman have a higher incidence of stress fractures compared with men. This difference is related to several factors, including lower BMD, nutritional issues, and menstrual irregularities. The association of disordered eating and menstrual disturbances with low BMD is not independent, but instead is interrelated. This relationship is termed the "female athlete triad" and is presented in a separate article.

MAKING THE DIAGNOSIS
History and Physical Examination

The typical history of a stress fracture is localized pain of insidious onset that is initially not present at the start but occurs toward the end of a run. If the athlete continues to run regularly, the pain typically occurs earlier in successive runs. A sign of a more advanced fracture is pain progressing to occur during non-running related activities, affecting day-to-day ambulation.

It is important to elucidate any predisposing factors while interviewing the runner with a suspected stress fracture. These questions include those regarding bone health (prior fractures, diet assessment and risk for disordered eating, menstrual history and current status in female runners), and specifics regarding training patterns. What changes in training have occurred? Has there been an increase in frequency, intensity, or distance of runs? Is the runner getting adequate rest from intense training? Has there been a recent change in running surface, technique, or shoes? Answers to these questions may provide opportunities for intervention.

The hallmark physical examination finding is focal bony tenderness. Overlying swelling, erythema, or warmth are other potential examination findings. Less sensitive tests for fractures of long bones include the fulcrum test and hop test. A functional kinetic chain assessment is useful to elucidate more subtle biomechanical factors that may predispose the runner to injury. Evaluating muscle imbalances; leg-length discrepancies; foot mechanics (pes cavus or planus); genu varum; and femoral anteversion is appropriate because all have been associated with stress fractures.[12,13]

Imaging

Radiographic imaging should be used to supplement the clinical history and physical examination in times of uncertainty (to confirm the diagnosis of stress fracture or rule out another source for symptoms) or when counseling a competitive runner who desires to continue training and requires confirmation. Imaging can also be used to grade the severity of injury and thus can be helpful in guiding treatment.

Plain radiography has rather low sensitivity for stress fracture, particularly in the first 2 weeks of symptoms. Often plain films are negative; however, an early radiographic sign is subtle periosteal bone formation. Other findings include a poorly defined cortical margin, osteopenia, and a discreet fracture line in severe cases. After the first few weeks, a visible callus is the most common finding of a healing fracture **Fig. 1**.

Radionuclide bone scintigraphy has high sensitivity but low specificity for stress fracture, however, there are cases of false negative examinations.[14,15] Abnormal findings can be seen within 6 to 72 hours of symptom onset.[13] The triple phase technique includes the immediate blood flow phase; the blood pool (or soft tissue) phase 1 to 5 minutes after injection; and the delayed (or skeletal) phase 3 to 6 hours post injection. Acute stress fractures are evident on all three phases. As the bony injury heals, the blood flow phase returns to normal first, followed by the blood pool phase a few weeks later. The findings on delayed imaging resolve last because of ongoing bony remodeling and commonly lag beyond the resolution of pain.[16] Soft-tissue injury is characterized by increased uptake in only the first two phases.

CT has little value in the routine evaluation of a runner with a suspected bony stress injury. CT is best used to differentiate lesions seen on bone scan that may mimic stress fracture, including osteoid osteoma, osteomyelitis, and malignancy. Its utility is also in differentiating a stress reaction from a true fracture by readily visualizing the fracture line, which can be particularly helpful in determining treatment in certain fractures (eg, pars inter-articularis or navicular).[17]

MRI is becoming the imaging study of choice, with many considering MRI the gold standard for the evaluation of bony stress injuries **Fig. 2**.[18] The advantages of MRI

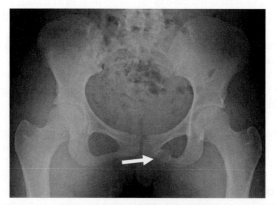

Fig. 1. Inferior pubic ramus fracture in a 14-year-old female basketball player at initial presentation 7 months after symptom onset. Note exuberant callous formation, likely caused by her young age and her continued play over that 7-month period before presentation.

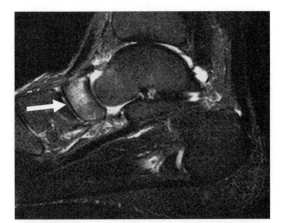

Fig. 2. Sagittal STIR MR image of a navicular stress reaction in a 42-year-old male recreational runner. No fracture line was noted on this MRI or subsequent CT.

include no ionizing radiation; the ability to visualize soft tissue (as a potential other source of pain); and its utility in visualizing bony edema consistent with a stress reaction. Its drawback is that not all stress reactions seen on MRI relate to clinical symptoms. Forty-three percent of 21 asymptomatic runners who were followed for 12 months in one study demonstrated evidence of stress injury on MRI of the tibia.[19] Fat suppression techniques, including short tau inversion recovery (STIR) and fat-suppressed T2-weighted images, maximize the sensitivity of MRI in detecting bone stress injuries. Fredericson and colleagues[20] have developed an MR grading system of tibial stress injuries that assists in guiding treatment and return to running (**Box 1**). In this study, runners with a grade 1 injury were able to return to soft-surface running within 2 to 3 weeks. Those with grade 2 injuries returned to running within 4 to 6 weeks, whereas the runners with grade 3 injuries returned to running in 6 to 9 weeks. The single runner with a grade 4 injury was treated with a cast for 6 weeks followed by a 6-week period of non-impact activities. Thus, MRI assists in planning treatment and counseling runners, but does demand an experienced diagnostician to decrease false-positive injuries.[21]

GENERAL TREATMENT PRINCIPLES

In guiding treatment, it is not only important to understand the significance of protection and rest but also to understand the predisposing factors to the injury. Treatment is the time to explore and treat the contributing risk factors. If there is a history of stress

---

Box 1
MRI grading of tibial stress injuries

Grade 1: Periosteal edema on fat-suppressed T2 images (shin splints)

Grade 2: Grade 1 + marrow edema on fat-suppressed T2 images

Grade 3: Grade 2 + marrow edema on T1 images

Grade 4: Grade 3 + clearly visible fracture line

Data from Fredericson M, Bergman AG, Hoffman KL, et al. Tibial stress reaction in runners correlation of clinical symptoms and scintigraphy with new magnetic resonance imaging grading system. Am J Sports Med 1995;23(4):472–81.

fracture or the fracture is of cancellous bone, a BMD assessment is indicated. If low bone density is found, appropriate treatment of the source (energy balance and nutritional issues or metabolic bone disease) is mandatory. Determining what training, shoe wear, or biomechanical issues are related will allow an appropriate individualized treatment program to include counseling the runner on how to more effectively train and providing specific rehabilitation guidelines once the runner is ready to return to training.

In general, the severity of the fracture and pain dictate how quickly a runner can progress back to regular training. Certain high-risk fractures require special treatment, which is discussed later in this article, according to the specific fracture location. For most fractures, relative rest from running is first and foremost. If there is pain with ambulation, then crutch walking or a limited period of non-weight bearing is indicated. Other options for pain control include ice and oral analgesics. Often times stopping the offending activity (running) is all that is necessary to control pain.

The rate of activity resumption is dependent on the severity of the fracture and the premorbid functional level of the runner. Activity should always be pain free; however, if pain should recur, the activity should cease for at least 1 to 2 days and then resume at a lower level. The runner should be pain free for approximately 2 weeks before returning to run training. During this time, all activities of daily living should be pain free and there should be no bony tenderness. **Table 1** demonstrates a typical return-to-running program for a non-elite athlete after the initial period of rest with an uncomplicated lower limb stress fracture.

Ultrasound and electrical stimulation are purported modalities for enhancing the healing rate of fractures. Therapeutic ultrasound has been demonstrated to decrease healing time in acute tibial shaft and distal radius fractures but not necessarily in stress fractures.[22,23] Using electrical stimulation for bone growth has some support in delayed unions and nonunions, but only in uncontrolled trials for stress fractures.[24]

There is one report of intravenous pamidronate used successfully to return five female collegiate basketball players with tibial fatigue fractures to play more quickly.[25] Bisphosphonates are commonly used in the treatment of postmenopausal osteoporosis. Bisphosphonates have demonstrated teratogenic effects in animal models. Because bisphosphonates remain in bone for years after administration, their use in pre-menopausal women may pose a teratogenic risk; though there have been no specific human reports.[26] Until large well-controlled studies of bisphosphonate use in premenopausal women are performed, their use should be limited in this population.

Table 1
Recreational (non-elite) return-to-running training program

	1	2	3	4	5	6	7
Week 1[a]	5 min	[b]	10 min	[b]	15 min	[b]	[b]
Week 2[a]	15 min	[b]	20 min	[b]	25 min	[b]	[b]
Week 3	25 min	30 min	[b]	30 min	35 min	40 min	[b]
Week 4	45 min	[c]	—	—	—	—	—

[a] Runs should occur on softer surfaces during the initial return-to-running phase.
[b] Non-impact activity on off days, which can be the same form of cross-training that the athlete was performing before resuming running.
[c] Gradual increase in distance and intensity depending on the runner's goals over weeks 4 to 6.

PREVENTING DECONDITIONING

Maintaining fitness during treatment of a lower-limb stress fracture is of significant concern to the running athlete. There are multiple non-weight–bearing methods to maintain cardiovascular fitness. These methods include cycling, swimming, deep-water running, and gravity-eliminated running. For the less competitive athlete, cycling and swimming may be adequate to maintain some form of aerobic fitness. However, for the competitive athlete, it is important to abide by the principle of sport specificity (ie, to train in the sport that the athlete competes to maintain or develop appropriate neuromuscular recruitment patterns). Deep-water running with a flotation device is an effective form of cross-training for the injured runner. During 4- to 8-week deep-water run training programs, runners maintained VO2max, anaerobic threshold, leg strength, and 2 mile and 5K run performance.[27,28] Antigravity treadmills, though costly, are gaining popularity in some universities and elite running programs to keep runners training while injured or to decrease injury risk in high-volume runners.

HIGH RISK STRESS FRACTURES
Femoral Neck

Femoral neck stress fracture is an infrequent, but important injury in the runners. Diagnosis is frequently delayed and serious complications are common. The exact incidence in competitive and recreational runners is difficult to determine. In a series of 1049 stress fractures occurring in athletes, femoral neck stress fractures represented 5%.[29] Some authors suggest that femoral neck stress fractures may represent an even higher percentage of stress fractures in athletes because of under diagnosis.[30]

The femoral neck is subjected to loading forces several times body weight and withstands considerable tensile and compressive forces. It is important to consider these two distinct forces separately because they lead to different injury types and outcomes. Tensile forces occur at the superior aspect of the femoral neck, whereas compressive forces occur at the inferior aspect.[31] Tension side femoral neck stress fractures are at higher risk for nonunion and displacement.[29,30,32] Other biomechanical factors, such as leg length inequality, coxa vara, and pes cavus, may also be important in the development of compressive and tensile injuries at the femoral neck.[7,13,32,33]

Runners with a history of anterior hip or groin pain worsened with activity. The pain has insidious onset and is often related to a change in type or intensity of workouts.[32] It is often difficult to illicit pain with palpation; however, pain may be present at the extremes of motion, with active straight leg raise, with log rolling, or with hopping.[29,34] Differential diagnosis contains many important entities in neoplastic, vascular, and musculoskeletal categories.

Many authors have demonstrated that plain radiographs will not reveal evidence of fracture in the first weeks following injury. This finding is particularly problematic given the high risk for fracture completion or displacement (**Fig. 3**). For this reason, it is generally recommended to proceed to MRI or bone scintigraphy when index of suspicion is high and plain radiographs are negative.[34] MRI is they study of choice as it allows for the early detection of marrow edema and stress reaction and is also a useful tool to screen for other causes of hip and groin pain.

Femoral neck stress fracture has many associated complications such as nonunion, malunion, osteonecrosis, and arthritic changes.[32,35] These complications may occur more frequently in the setting of a displaced fracture.[36] Johansson and colleagues[35] have reported a 30% complication rate in a series of athletes with femoral neck stress fracture. Similarly, in a series of 12 femoral neck stress fractures treated surgically by Visuri and colleagues,[36] seven subjects developed osteonecrosis, delayed union, or

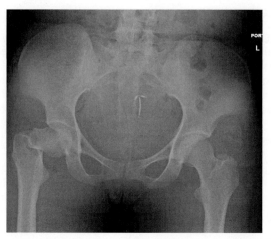

Fig. 3. Displaced femoral neck fracture in a 22-year-old woman with a history of treatment for anorexia. Her symptoms presented at mile 10 during a marathon. She initially noted right groin pain while running at mile 10, stopped to "stretch it out," then resumed running. Within a half mile she collapsed to the ground. She was transferred to a local hospital and underwent immediate open reduction internal fixation.

nonunion. In the young active population, progression to avascular necrosis has been reported in 20% to 86% of cases by various authors.[37,38]

Treatment is based on the anatomic location of the fracture. Many authors suggest that tension side femoral neck stress fractures require internal fixation because of potential instability and high rate of complications; however, there are reports of successful conservative management for non-displaced tension side fractures.[29] Compression side fractures are generally treated conservatively with a period of rest followed by gradual return to activity and exercises. Femoral neck stress fractures treated conservatively should have frequent radiographic monitoring for progression given the high incidence. Return to running is considered when full weight bearing is asymptomatic, there is no tenderness to palpation on physical examination, and imaging studies are consistent with healed fracture.

Anterior Tibia

Stress fracture of the anterior tibia is a common high-risk stress fracture in athletes and should always be considered in the runner with anterior leg pain. Tibial stress fractures in general account for nearly 50% of stress fractures in athletes[13,39]; however, the majority of these are posteromedial in nature and considered low risk.[40] Anterior tibial fractures occur on the tension side of the bone and are considered to be at higher risk for delayed healing and nonunion.

In the case of anterior stress fractures, patients may have little symptomatic discomfort even in the setting of nonunion.[41] Patients may also describe anterior leg pain or vague discomfort. A history of training regime change is often appreciated. Physical examination may reveal localized tenderness to palpation, swelling, or palpable callus.[40] Differential diagnosis includes medial tibial stress syndrome (MTSS); stress reaction; muscle strain; neoplasm; and exertional compartment syndrome. Though often difficult to delineate on the basis of history and physical examination, pain from a tibial stress fracture may be distinguished from medial tibial stress syndrome based on persistence of symptoms at rest and with daily ambulation. Another defining difference is that MTSS rarely causes proximal tibial pain.[42]

Workup with initial plain radiographs is appropriate; however, progression to more advanced imaging studies is recommended if repeat radiographs remain negative after 2 to 3 weeks of continued symptoms. Plain film findings include periosteal reaction and anterior fracture line, commonly referred to as the "dreaded black line." Bone scan has traditionally been the gold standard, but recent data suggest that MRI is more specific, has greater usefulness for grading purposes, and can detect pre-fracture stress reactions.[19,43]

Treatment of an anterior tibial stress fracture involves surgical referral with consideration of intramedullary nailing. Varner followed seven college athletes with chronic mid-tibial stress fractures failing conservative management and ultimately treated with intramedullary nailing.[44] Radiological union occurred on average at 3 months with return to play occurring at an average of 4 months. These and other authors suggest that intramedullary nailing allows for earlier return to play in athletic populations. There have also been several series suggesting conservative treatment with rest, and pneumatic bracing may be effective in healing anterior tibial stress fractures with return to full participation occurring at approximately 8 months post diagnosis.[24,45]

Medial Malleolus

Stress fractures of the medial malleolus are infrequent but can occur in runners and other athletes. They account for 0.6% to 4.1% of all stress fractures and are significantly less common than fractures at the distal fibula and lateral malleolus.[39,46]

The pathogenesis of medial malleolus stress fractures is related to abnormal weight transmission and torsional forces without a significant role for muscular forces.[46] It has been postulated that closed chain loading during stance leads to a series of biomechanical events with ultimate transmission of force to the medial malleolus.[47] Abnormal weight transmission, small angle between the tibial shaft and plafond, and tibia vara alignment have all been suggested as possible risk factors for stress fracture of the medial malleolus.[48,49]

Patients typically present with pain of insidious onset with strong localization to the medial malleolus. Pain generally begins after change in exercise regimen or intensity. On examination, patients are often tender to palpation and effusion may be present.[46] Differential diagnosis includes neoplasm, infection, ankle sprain, tendonitis, compartment syndrome, tendon tear, and shin splints.

Plain radiographs are often initially negative and may not show evidence of fracture for 2 to 4 weeks.[47–50] Medial malleolus stress fractures have been described as vertical fractures occurring at the junction of the medial malleolus and tibial plafond and extending proximally.[42] MRI is a sensitive and useful tool for the diagnosis of this injury.[48]

Treatment is generally conservative. A Pneumatic brace is typically recommended for 6 weeks in non-displaced or minimally displaced stress fractures of the medial malleolus.[47] Complete rest is to be avoided given the potential for atrophy and deconditioning.[42] For displaced fractures, open reduction and internal fixation with screws is recommended, with generally good outcomes reported.[47–49]

Navicular

Navicular stress fractures are common and have been reported to account for up to 15% to 30% of all stress fractures.[51,52] The great majority of these fractures appear to occur in track and field athletes, such has jumpers, hurdlers, sprinters, and middle distance runners, as opposed to long-distance runners.[7] Navicular stress fracture is also more common in men.[53]

The anatomic location and the vascular supply of the navicular bone lead to its vulnerability. Compression between the talus and cuneiforms during heel strike leads to focused force on the central third of the bone.[54] Additionally, the central portion of the navicular has a relative decrease in vascular supply leading to further vulnerability and potential for poor healing.[55] Numerous biomechanical factors for navicular stress fracture have also been postulated, including pes cavus, short first metatarsal, metatarsus adductus, limited subtalar or ankle motion, and medial narrowing of the talonavicular joint; however, true significance of these factors remains unclear.[55–57]

Patients with navicular stress fracture generally report insidious onset of pain with increased pain after activities.[58] Pain is in the midfoot and may localize more specifically to the navicular as the injury progresses.[55,57] The pain may be aggravated with specific movement, such as jumping and pushing off, and often subsides quickly following periods of rest.[57–59] Commonly, a recent increase in training or change to training regimen is reported. Physical examination may reveal tenderness over the navicular bone, particularly at the dorsal aspect or "N Spot." Pain may be reproducible with push-off maneuvers or jumping.

The diagnosis can be made with plain radiographs; however, images may be normal for 3 to 6 weeks.[60] Bone scan has been used to assist in ruling out navicular stress fracture because of high sensitivity.[61] CT scan is highly effective in diagnosing navicular stress fracture.[17] MRI is increasingly recommended because of high sensitivity, particularly with regard to detecting early changes that may lead to earlier treatment.[60,62]

Because of its multifactorial vulnerability as discussed earlier, navicular stress fracture is considered to be at high risk for complications, such as delayed union and nonunion. Stress fracture of the navicular bone has a particularly high rate of failure when treated with decreased activity, but continued weight bearing.[63] For this reason patients must wear a non-weight–bearing cast until the fracture is healed. Saxena has proposed categorization of navicular fracture into three types to guide surgical intervention.[63] Type 1 fractures, involving the dorsal cortex only, can be trialed in a non-weight–bearing cast for 6 weeks. Types 2 and 3 (break into the navicular body and the opposite cortex, respectively) require surgical intervention. This intervention usually consists of percutaneous fixation, with bone grafting used in the case of chronic fracture, delayed union, or non-union.

Rehabilitation includes a graduated progression once the cast is removed and is guided by pain with weight bearing and tenderness at the N-Spot. Patients may require up to 8 months for return to previous level of activity.[64] In Khan's and colleagues[63] study of 55 subjects with navicular stress fracture, 86% were able to return to full activity in an average of 5.6 months when treated non-operatively with 6 weeks of a non-weight–bearing cast. In the series by Saxena and colleagues,[64] subjects with type 1, 2, and 3 navicular stress fractures returned to full activity in an average of 3.0, 3.6, and 6.8 months, respectively.

Proximal Fifth Metatarsal

Stress fracture of the proximal fifth metatarsal is a rare, but important fracture in runners given its high rate of delayed healing and nonunion. In the athletic population in general, metatarsal stress fracture represents 9% to 19% of stress fractures with the second and third metatarsal shafts accounting for 80% of these fractures.[13,65] In a review of 204 march fractures in German soldiers, 89% of stress fractures occurred in the second and third metatarsals with only 11% occurring in the first, fourth, and fifth combined.[66]

Multiple series have demonstrated 20% to 67% nonunion rates in proximal fifth metatarsal fractures.[67,68] The blood supply to this bone is the major factor in the high rate of delayed or nonunion. There is a potential watershed area between the metaphyseal perforating arteries and the terminal branches of the nutrient arteries. This watershed area correlates with the zone of poor fracture healing reported.[65,69] Proximal fifth metatarsal fractures are classified into three zones.[67,70] Zone one fractures correspond to the most proximal region of the fifth metatarsal and typically occur as avulsion fractures, often with acute inversion of the foot.[71] Zone two fractures occur at the metaphyseal-diaphysis junction and are classically referred to as "Jones" fractures. They are thought to occur when adduction forces are applied to the forefoot while the ankle is plantar flexed. Zone three fractures refer to fractures of the proximal 1.5cm of the diaphysis. These fractures are considered to be true stress fractures, occurring when repetitive forces outweigh bone remodeling capacity.[65] Zone three stress fractures may predispose the athlete to acute zone one and zone two fractures.[68]

Runners typically report a change in running regimen or a history of acute trauma. Pain with weight bearing is the most common symptom. There may be tenderness to palpation, swelling, and ecchymosis. In the setting of acute fracture, plain radiographs often lead to the diagnosis, but are often negative in the initial workup of stress fractures. With high index of suspicion, MRI or bone scan should be considered given the potential for complication and progression as described earlier.

Treatment for acute non-displaced Jones fractures and diaphyseal stress fractures is generally 6 to 8 weeks of non-weight–bearing ambulation in a short leg cast. Partial weight-bearing strategies have demonstrated higher rates of delayed union.[65,70,71] In the case of a high-performance athlete, early surgical intervention can be considered.[71,72] For patients with displaced and widened fractures, or continued symptoms despite conservative management, surgical consultation should be obtained. Multiple open and closed surgical interventions exist with mean time to radiographic healing in approximately 8 weeks.[73,74]

Sesamoids

Sesamoid stress fractures represent approximately 1% to 3% of stress fractures in athletes.[13,39] They are important injuries to consider in runners with forefoot pain given the potential for complications, such as delayed union and nonunion, and thus, often require surgical intervention.

The sesamoid bones function as a pulley for the flexor hallucis longus and brevis tendons and provide stabilization at the metatarsophalangeal (MTP) joint. This unique biomechanical position leads to repetitive stress and potential for fracture.

In a series of five athletes, swelling at the forefoot and activity-related pain that increased in forced dorsiflexion, but disappeared at rest, were found in all subjects with sesamoid stress fracture.[75] Other series have described the insidious onset of pain at the first MTP joint during athletic activity.[76] Physical examination may also reveal tenderness to palpation over the sesamoids. Other causes of sesamoid pain include acute fractures, nonunions, osteonecrosis, chondromalacia, and sesamoiditis. Forefoot pain and metatarsalgia in general has a fairly expansive differential.

As in most stress fractures, initial radiographs are often negative. Stress fracture may be difficult to diagnosis in the setting of bipartite or multipartite sesamoid complexes. With high clinical suspicion, or in the setting of multipartite sesamoids, additional imaging in the form of bone scan or MRI should be pursued.

Sesamoid stress fractures are at high risk for delayed union, nonunion, osteonecrosis, and sesamoiditis. For this reason, a prolonged period of non-weight–bearing or casting with clinical and radiographic monitoring before return to activity is recommended.[76] Once symptom free, the runner can gradually begin rehabilitation. If conservative treatment with casting for at least 6 weeks fails to relieve tenderness and pain with weight bearing, most authors agree that sesamoidectomy should be considered. Multiple series investigating return to play following sesamoidectomy demonstrate successful symptom-free return to play at an average of 10 weeks postoperative.[76,77]

LOW RISK STRESS FRACTURES
Sacrum

Sacral stress fracture is an important diagnosis to consider because it often mimics other causes of back and gluteal-region pain, but requires a much different approach to treatment. The exact incidence of sacral stress fractures in runners is unknown; however, there have been multiple case reports and series describing this injury.[78–80] The sacrum serves as the keystone in the arch of the pelvis and is subject to multiple forces that may cause stress fracture. Patients generally have nonspecific complaints of lower back and buttock pain. Plain radiographs generally do not lead to the diagnosis. MRI may reveal linear abnormal signal intensity paralleling the sacroiliac joint, whereas CT may reveal linear sclerosis with cortical disruption. Bone scan reveals increased uptake that typically parallels the sacroiliac joint. There is no clear consensus for the optimal study; however, MRI appears to provide increased detail regarding anatomic location.[81] Treatment regimens in the reported cases have generally consisted of 6 to 8 weeks of rest followed by gradual return to activity once symptom free. Knobloch and colleagues[82] have outlined a progressive rehabilitation program for the long-distance runner.

Pubic Ramus

Stress fractures of the pelvis account for roughly 1% to 7% of all stress fractures, and most commonly occur at the inferior pubic ramus.[42,83] A high percentage of the pubic ramus stress fractures reported in athletes occur in long-distance runners.[83,84] Stress fractures at this anatomic site are thought to result from repetitive tensile stresses of the adductor magnus at its origin on the inferior pubic ramus.[85] Patients may present with groin pain that is initially often mistaken for an adductor strain. There have been informal reports of pubic ramus stress fractures requiring extended periods of rest, including non-weight–bearing. Because relative rest may not be sufficient, early diagnosis is essential. As in the stress fractures previously presented, negative plain radiographs in the setting of high clinical suspicion, warrant further study with bone scan or MRI. Weight bearing and ultimate return to sport should be guided by pain. A period of non-weight bearing, though not common, may be necessary to heal stress fractures of the pubic ramus.

Femoral Shaft

Femoral shaft stress fractures are considered low risk compared with stress fracture of the femoral neck. Stress fracture of the femoral shaft represents approximately 3% to 20% of stress fractures in athletes and is considered to be an under-diagnosed injury. In athletic populations, this injury most commonly occurs in the mid-medial and posteromedial cortex.[86,87] Fractures in these areas are largely caused by compressive forces. The compressive strain on the medial side of the femur is greater than the lateral tensile strain. The point of highest strain occurs in the posterior proximal shaft.[88] Patients generally present with insidious onset of pain that is nonspecific and localized in the groin, thigh, or knee. Pain with palpation at a particular area is less likely given the overlying muscle bulk of the thigh. A broad differential should be considered given the often vague presentation. As in most stress fractures, early diagnosis requires the use of MRI or bone scan as opposed to plain radiography. Patients with femoral shaft stress fractures require a comprehensive assessment of risk factors and are generally treated conservatively. Return to play is approached gradually and is guided by pain with weight bearing and activity. Ivkovic and colleagues[89] have proposed a treatment and rehabilitation algorithm for femoral shaft fractures in athletes.

Tibia

Stress fractures in runners occur most commonly at the tibia. Tibial stress fractures account for nearly 50% of all stress fractures in athletes.[13] The majority of these fractures occur at the posteromedial aspect of the middle third of the tibial shaft, which is considered a site of low risk for complication. Other higher-risk sites of the tibia, such as the anterior cortex and medial malleolus, are discussed earlier. Stress fracture of the tibia should be suspected in any athlete with leg pain that is worsened with weight bearing and exercise. Differentiating the source of medial shin pain in the runner, on the continuum of medial tibial stress syndrome to overt stress fracture, is often difficult. Plain radiographs are typically normal in the setting of early tibial stress fracture and MRI or bone scan may be required to reveal stress fractures and early stress reactions. Treatment and return to play should be considered on an individual basis in the case of low-risk tibial stress fractures and can be guided by pain-free weight-bearing activity. Pneumatic bracing is effective adjunct in the treatment of these fractures.[5] A rest period of 2 to 6 weeks is generally recommended, followed by low-impact exercise and gradual return to previous level of function.[40] It may take several months for runners to return to prior workout intensity. If symptoms persist or fractures progress, surgical intervention may be necessary. Some authors advocate early fixation with intramedullary nailing to allow earlier return to play in high-level athletes.

Fibula

Though the exact incidence in runners is uncertain, fibular stress fractures account for 4.6% to 21% of all stress fractures in athletes.[39,47,48] Fibular stress fractures most commonly occur at the distal third of the fibula. Burrows[90] noted that stress fractures occurring 5 to 6 cm proximal to the lateral malleolus occur more frequently in young male athletes. These fractures are referred to as "runner's fractures" and occur at narrow cortical bone as opposed to the cancellous bone of the malleolus itself. Middle-aged women were more likely to have stress fractures 3 to 4 cm from the lateral malleolus, occurring in cancellous bone. Because the fibula has less of a role in weight bearing, muscular forces have been implicated in the development of fibular stress fractures. Contractions of the ankle plantar flexors in runners are thought to approximate the fibula to the tibia, with resultant stress concentration at the runner's fracture site. More distal fractures occurring at the lateral malleolus may be related to osteoporosis and intrinsic bone quality given the tendency for these fractures to occur in middle-aged women.[91] Patients generally present with pain near the area of fracture and will often describe a recent change in exercise intensity. As in most stress fractures, initial radiographs may be negative, necessitating the use of MRI or bone scan to establish the diagnosis. Conservative treatment is generally appropriate for fibular stress fractures and is similar to that described for other low-risk stress fractures.

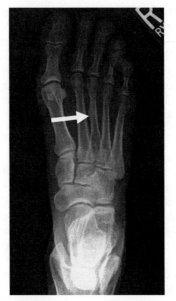

Fig. 4. Typical location of a mid-shaft metatarsal stress fracture in a 41-year-old female elite triathlete. Note callous formation 6 weeks after initial injury. Her initial symptoms presented while doing interval training on the track 4 days after winning a sprint distance race.

Metatarsal Shaft

Stress fractures of the metatarsals are common, especially in runners, and represent approximately 10% to 20% of stress fractures among athletes.[13] Of metatarsal stress fractures, 80% occur in the second and third metatarsal shaft. High-risk fractures of the proximal fifth metatarsal are separately discussed in this article. Metatarsal stress fractures; often referred to as "march fractures," frequently occur with a change in running regimen or intensity. Patients typically describe pain with activity and may be able to indicate a localized point of tenderness. Evaluation of suspected metatarsal shaft fractures should include plain radiographs with MRI or bone scan in the setting of negative radiographs and high index of suspicion **Fig. 4**. Treatment of non-displaced metatarsal shaft stress fractures is nonoperative and often uses a hard-sole postoperative shoe, a prefabricated walker boot, or a short-leg cast with progressive weight bearing for 4 to 6 weeks.[66] Gradual rehabilitation and return to activity is recommended.

REFERENCES

1. Pepper M, Akuthota V, McCarty EC. The pathophysiology of stress fractures. Clin Sports Med 2006;25:1–16.
2. Johanson MA. Contributing factors in microtrauma injuries of the lower extremity. J Back Musculoskelet Rehabil 1992;2:12–25.
3. Milgrom C, Firestone A, Segev, et al. Are overground or treadmill runners more likely to sustain tibial stress fracture? Br J Sports Med 2003;37(2):160–3.
4. Gardner LI, Dziados JE, Jones BH, et al. Prevention of lower extremity stress fractures: a controlled trial of shock absorbent insole. Am J Public Health 1988;78:1563–7.

5. Rome K, Handoll HHG, Ashford RL. Interventions for preventing and treating stress fractures and stress reactions of bone of the lower limbs in young adults. Cochrane Database Syst Rev 2005;2:CD000450.

6. Ekenman I, Milgrom C, Finestone A, et al. The role of biomechanical shoe orthoses in tibial stress fracture prevention. Am J Sports Med 2002;30(6): 866–70.

7. Bennell KL, Malcolm SA, Thomas SA, et al. The incidence and distribution of stress fractures in competitive track and field athletes: a twelve month prospective study. Am J Sports Med 1996;24(2):211–7.

8. Giladi M, Milgrom M, Simkin A, et al. Stress fractures and tibial bone width: a risk factor. J Bone Joint Surg Br 1987;69(2):326–9.

9. Bennell K, Crossley K, Jayarajan J, et al. Ground reaction forces and bone parameters in females with tibial stress fracture. Med Sci Sports Exerc 2004; 36:397–404.

10. Pohl MB, Mullineaux DR, Milner CE, et al. Biomechanical predictors of retrospective tibial stress fractures in runners. J Biomech 2008;41:1160–5.

11. Milner CE, Ferber R, Pollard C, et al. Biomechanical factors associated with tibial stress fracture in female runners. Med Sci Sports Exerc 2006;38(2):323–8.

12. James SL, Bates BT, Osternig LR. Injuries to runners. Am J Sports Med 1978;6: 40–50.

13. Matheson GO, Clement DB, McKenzie DC, et al. Stress fractures in athletes: a study of 320 cases. Am J Sports Med 1987;15(1):46–58.

14. Keen JS, Lash EG. Negative bone scan in a femoral neck stress fracture: a case report. Am J Sports Med 1992;20:234–6.

15. Sterling JC, Webb RF, Meyers MC, et al. False negative bone scan in a female runner. Med Sci Sports Exerc 1993;25:179–85.

16. Ammann W, Matheson GO. Radionuclide imaging in the detection of stress fractures. Clin J Sport Med 1991;1:115–22.

17. Kiss ZA, Khan KM, Fuller PJ. Stress fractures of the tarsal navicular bone: CT findings in 55 cases. AJR Am J Roentgenol 1993;160(1):111–5.

18. Kiuru MJ, Pihlajamaki HK, Hietanen HJ, et al. MR imaging, bone scintigraphy, and radiography in bone stress injuries of the pelvis and the lower extremity. Acta Radiol 2008;43(2):207–12.

19. Bergman AG, Fredericson M, Ho C, et al. Asymptomatic tibial stress reactions: MRI detection and clinical follow-up in distance runners. AJR Am J Roentgenol 2004;183:635–8.

20. Fredericson M, Bergman AG, Hoffman KL, et al. Tibial stress reaction in runners correlation of clinical symptoms and scintigraphy with new magnetic resonance imaging grading system. Am J Sports Med 1995;23(4):472–81.

21. Moran DS, Evans RK, Hadad E. Imaging of lower extremity stress fracture injuries. Sports Med 2008;38(4):345–56.

22. Heckman JD, Ryaby JP, McCabe J, et al. Acceleration of tibial fracture healing by non-invasive low-intensity pulsed ultrasound. J Bone Joint Surg Am 1994;76: 26–34.

23. Kristianson TK, Ryaby JP, McCabe J, et al. Accelerated healing of distal radial fractures with the use of specific, low-intensity ultrasound. A multicenter, prospective, randomized, double-blind, placebo-controlled trial. J Bone Joint Surg Am 1997;79:961–73.

24. Rettig AC, Shelbourne KD, McCarroll JR, et al. The natural history and treatment of delayed union stress fractures of the anterior cortex of the tibia. Am J Sports Med 1988;16:250–5.

25. Stewart GW, Brunet ME, Manning MR, et al. Treatment of stress fractures in athletes with intravenous pamidronate. Clin J Sport Med 2005;15:92–4.

26. McNicholl DM, Heaney LG. The safety of bisphosphonate use in pre-menopausal women on corticosteroids. Curr Drug Saf 2010. [Epub ahead of print].

27. Bushman BA, Flynn MG, Andres FF, et al. Effect of 4 wk of deep water run training on performance. Med Sci Sports Exerc 1997;29(5):694–9.

28. Wilbur RL, Moffatt RJ, Scott BE, et al. Influence of water run training on the maintenance of aerobic performance. Med Sci Sports Exerc 1996;28(8):1056–62.

29. Fullerton L, Snowdy H. Femoral neck stress fractures. Am J Sports Med 1988;16:365–77.

30. DeFranco MJ, Recht M, Schils J, et al. Stress fractures of the femur in athletes. Clin Sports Med 2006;25(1):89–103.

31. Egol KA, Koval KJ, Kummer F, et al. Stress fractures of the femoral neck. Clin Orthop Relat Res 1998;348:72–8.

32. Fullerton LR Jr. Femoral neck stress fractures. Sports Med 1990;9(3):192–7.

33. Tuan K, Wu S, Sennett B. Stress fractures in athletes: risk factors, diagnosis, and management. Orthopedics 2004;27:583–91.

34. Shin A, Mortin W, Gorman J, et al. The superiority of magnetic resonance imaging in differentiating the cause of hip pain in endurance athletes. Am J Sports Med 1996;24(2):168–76.

35. Johansson C, Ekenman I, Tornkvist H, et al. Stress fractures of the femoral neck in athletes. Am J Sports Med 1990;18:524–8.

36. Visuri T, Vara A, Meurman KO. Displaced stress fractures of the femoral neck in young male adults: a report of twelve operative cases. J Trauma 1988;28(11):1562–9.

37. Visuri T. Stress osteopathy of the femoral head. 10 military recruits followed for 5–11 years. Acta Orthop Scand 1997;68(2):138–41.

38. Lee C, Huang G, Chao K, et al. Surgical treatment of displaced stress fractures of the femoral neck in military recruits: a report of 42 cases. Arch Orthop Trauma Surg 2003;123:527–33.

39. Iwamoto J, Takeda T. Stress fractures in athletes: review of 196 cases. J Orthop Sci 2003;8:273–8.

40. Young AJ, McAllister DR. Evaluation and treatment of tibial stress fractures. Clin Sports Med 2006;25(1):117–28.

41. Bruckner P, Bennell K. Stress fractures. In: O'Connor F, Wilder R, editors. Textbook of running medicine. New York (NY): McGraw-Hill Professional; 2001. p. 227–56, Chapter 19.

42. Fredericson M, Jennings F, Beaulieu C, et al. Stress fractures in athletes. Top Magn Reson Imaging 2006;17(5):309–25.

43. Kiuru MJ, Niva M, Reponen A, et al. Bone stress injuries in asymptomatic elite recruits. Am J Sports Med 2005;33(2):272–6.

44. Varner KE, Younas SA, Lintner DM, et al. Chronic anterior midtibial stress fractures in athletes treated with reamed intramedullary nailing. Am J Sports Med 2005;33(7):1071–6.

45. Batt ME, Kemp S, Kerslake R. Delayed union stress fractures of the anterior tibia: conservative management. Br J Sports Med 2001;35(1):74–7.

46. Sherbondy PS. Stress fracture of the medial malleolus and distal fibula. Clin Sports Med 2006;25(1):129–37.

47. Shelbourne KD, Fisher DA, Rettig AC, et al. Stress fractures of the medial malleolus. Am J Sports Med 1988;16:60–3.

48. Orava S, Karpakka J, Taimela S, et al. Stress fracture of the medial malleolus. J Bone Joint Surg Am 1995;77A:362–5.
49. Kor A, Saltzman AT, Wempe PD. Medial malleolar stress fractures: literature review, diagnosis, and treatment. J Am Podiatr Med Assoc 2003;93:292–7.
50. Okada K, Senma S, Abe E, et al. Stress fractures of the medial malleolus: a case report. Foot Ankle Int 1995;16:49–52.
51. Brukner P, Bradshaw C, Khan KM, et al. Stress fractures: a review of 180 cases. Clin J Sport Med 1996;6:85–9.
52. Bennell K, Malcolm S, Thomas S, et al. Risk factors for stress fractures in track and field athletes. Am J Sports Med 1996;24:810–8.
53. Jones MH, Amendola AS. Navicular stress fractures. Clin Sports Med 2006;25(1): 151.
54. Van Langelaan EJ. A kinematic analysis of the tarsal joints: an x-ray photogrammetric study. Acta Orthop Scand Suppl 1983;204:1–269.
55. Golano P, Farinas O, Saenz I. The anatomy of the navicular and periarticular structures. Foot Ankle Clin 2004;9:1–23.
56. Pavlov H, Torg JS, Freiberger RH. Tarsal navicular stress fractures: radiographic evaluation. Radiology 1983;148:641–5.
57. Ting A, King W, Yocum L, et al. Stress fractures of the tarsal navicular in long-distance runners. Clin Sports Med 1988;7:89–101.
58. Fitch KD, Blackwell JB, Gilmour WN. Operation for non-union of stress fracture of the tarsal navicular. J Bone Joint Surg Br 1989;71:105–10.
59. Hunter LY. Stress fracture of the tarsal navicular. More frequent than we realize? Am J Sports Med 1981;9(4):217–9.
60. Sizensky JA, Marks RM. Imaging of the navicular. Foot Ankle Clin 2004;9: 181–209.
61. Mann JA, Pedowitz DI. Evaluation and treatment of navicular stress fractures, including nonunions, revision surgery, and persistent pain after treatment. Foot Ankle Clin 2009;14(2):187–204.
62. Burne SG, Mahoney CM, Forster BB, et al. Tarsal navicular stress injury: long-term outcome and clinicoradiological correlation using both computed tomography and magnetic resonance imaging. Am J Sports Med 2005;33:1875–81.
63. Khan KM, Fuller PJ, Brukner PD, et al. Outcome of conservative and surgical management of navicular stress fracture in athletes: eighty-six cases proven with computerized tomography. Am J Sports Med 1992;20:657–66.
64. Saxena A, Fullem B, Hannaford D. Results of treatment of 22 navicular stress fractures and a new proposed radiographic classification system. J Foot Ankle Surg 2000;39:96–103.
65. Fetzer GB, Wright RW. Metatarsal shaft fractures and fractures of the proximal fifth metatarsal. Clin Sports Med 2006;25(1):139–50.
66. Henningsen A, Hinz P, Lüdde R, et al. Retrospective analysis of march fractures in the german armed forces in the years 1998 to 2000. Z Orthop Ihre Grenzgeb 2006;144(5):502–6.
67. Dameron TB. Fractures of the proximal fifth metatarsal: selecting the best treatment option. J Am Acad Orthop Surg 1995;3(2):110–4.
68. Kavanaugh JH, Brower TD, Mann RV. The Jones fracture revisited. J Bone Joint Surg Am 1978;60:776–82.
69. Smith JW, Arnoczky SP, Hersh A. The interosseous blood supply of the fifth metatarsal: implications for proximal fracture healing. Foot Ankle 1992;13(3):143–52.
70. Lawrence SJ, Botte MJ. Jones' fractures and related fractures of the proximal fifth metatarsal. Foot Ankle 1993;14:358–65.

71. Rosenberg GA, Sferra JJ. Treatment strategies for acute fractures and nonunions of the proximal fifth metatarsal. J Am Acad Orthop Surg 2000;8(5):332–8.

72. Nunley JA. Fractures of the base of the fifth metatarsal: the Jones fracture. Orthop Clin North Am 2001;32(1):171–80.

73. Larson CM, Almekinders LC, Taft TN, et al. Intramedullary screw fixation of Jones fractures. Analysis of failure. Am J Sports Med 2002;30(1):55–60.

74. Porter DA, Duncan M, Meyer SJ. Fifth metatarsal Jones fracture fixation with a 4.5-mm cannulated stainless steel screw in the competitive and recreational athlete. A clinical and radiographic evaluation. Am J Sports Med 2005;33(5):1–8.

75. Biedert R, Hintermann B. Stress fractures of the medial great toe sesamoids in athletes. Foot Ankle Int 2003;24(2):137–41.

76. Van Hal ME, Keene JS, Lange TA. Stress fractures of the great toe sesamoids. Am J Sports Med 1982;10(2):122–8.

77. Saxena A, Krisdakumtorn T. Return to activity after sesamoidectomy in athletically active individuals. Foot Ankle Int 2003;24(5):415–9.

78. Alsobrook J, Simons SM. Sacral stress fracture in a female collegiate distance runner: a case report. Curr Sports Med Rep 2007;6(1):39–42.

79. Fredericson M, Salamancha L, Bealieu C. Sacral stress fractures, tracking nonspecific pain in distance runners. Phys Sportsmed 2003;31(2):31–42.

80. Shah MK, Stewart GW. Sacral stress fractures: an unusual cause of low back pain in an athlete. Spine 2002;27(4):104–8.

81. Major N, Helms C. Sacral stress fractures in long-distance runners. Am J Roentgenol 2000;174:727–9.

82. Knobloch K, Schreibmueller L, Jagodzinski M, et al. Rapid rehabilitation programme following sacral stress fracture in a long-distance running female athlete. Arch Orthop Trauma Surg 2007;127:809–13.

83. Hosey RG, Fernandez MM, Johnson DL. Evaluation and management of stress fractures of the pelvis and sacrum. Orthopedics 2008;31(4):383–5.

84. Kiuru MJ, Pihlajamaki HK, Ahovuo JA. Fatigue stress injuries of the pelvic bones and proximal femur: evaluation with MR imaging. Eur Radiol 2003;13:605–11.

85. Ha KI, Hahn SH, Chung MY, et al. A clinical study of stress fractures in sports activities. Orthopedics 1991;14(10):1089–95.

86. Hershman E, Lombardo J, Bergfeld J. Femoral shaft stress fractures in athletes. Am J Sports Med 1990;9:111–9.

87. Johnson A, Weiss C, Wheeler D. Stress fractures of the femoral shaft in athletes: more common than expected. Am J Sports Med 1994;22:248–56.

88. Oh I, Harris W. Proximal strain distribution in the loaded femur. J Bone Joint Surg Am 1978;60A:75–85.

89. Ivkovic A, Bojanic I, Pecina M. Stress fractures of the femoral shaft in athletes: a new treatment algorithm. Br J Sports Med 2006;40:518–20.

90. Burrows HJ. Fatigue fractures of the fibula. J Bone Joint Surg Br 1948;30B:266–79.

91. Miller MD, Marks PH, Fu FH. Bilateral stress fractures of the distal fibula in a 35-year-old woman. Foot Ankle Int 1994;15:450–3.

Running and Osteoarthritis

Stuart E. Willick, MD*, Pamela A. Hansen, MD

KEYWORDS

• Running • Osteoarthritis • Sports epidemiology
• Articular cartilage

Running has many benefits.[1] It can be personally and socially rewarding. Running has been shown to improve cardiovascular endurance and help control blood pressure and levels of lipids and cholesterol.[2] Running is a useful form of weight management and can improve strength, endurance, and mood.[2,3]

Yet running is not without risk. Running overload injuries to muscle, tendon, and bone are common. Less well understood, however, is the relationship between running and joint injury. Where is the balance between running for fun and health promotion versus injury risk? The sports medicine practitioner frequently hears runners ask if they can do permanent damage to their joints if they continue running. This is a logical question because all mechanical devices eventually break down with repetitive loading. However, biologic joints differ from nonbiologic mechanical constructions in that they possess intrinsic healing mechanisms designed to combat the inevitable breakdown process. It is plausible that repetitive loading of joints during running may favor the breakdown process. It is also possible, however, that running might stimulate joint health and joint healing.[1]

This article reviews the available literature on the association between running and the development of osteoarthritis. Serving as background, the first part of the article briefly reviews the clinical, histologic, and radiologic findings of osteoarthritis. The second part summarizes in vitro and human epidemiologic studies that offer theoretical considerations regarding the relationship between running and osteoarthritis. The third section covers in vivo animal studies. The final and perhaps most clinically relevant section examines in vivo human studies that explore the association between running and the development of osteoarthritis.

OSTEOARTHRITIS

Osteoarthritis is the most common form of joint disease. It is characterized by degeneration of the articular cartilage, with eburnation of subchondral bone and hypertrophy

Neither author has any financial disclosures.
Division of Physical Medicine and Rehabilitation, University of Utah Orthopaedic Center, 590 Wakara Way, Salt Lake City, UT 84108, USA
* Corresponding author.
E-mail address: stuart.willick@hsc.utah.edu

Clin Sports Med 29 (2010) 417–428
doi:10.1016/j.csm.2010.03.006
0278-5919/10/$ – see front matter © 2010 Elsevier Inc. All rights reserved.

of bone at the articular margins resulting in osteophyte formation.[4] Osteoarthritis may be classified as primary (idiopathic) or secondary. Secondary osteoarthritis has many causes, including trauma; damage from other inflammatory diseases; and developmental anomalies such as malalignment, hip dysplasia, and hip impingement morphology.

Osteoarthritis usually has an insidious onset and follows a slow progressive course. The clinical findings include joint stiffness, variable pain that is worsened by use and weight bearing, deformity, limitation of motion, crepitus, and synovitis or other signs of local inflammation without systemic manifestations. Radiologic findings of osteoarthritis include joint space narrowing, osteophyte formation, intra-articular osseous bodies, subchondral sclerosis, and subchondral cysts.[5] The physical findings often do not correlate with the radiographic findings. Sometimes people have marked degenerative joint changes on radiographs with minimal or no symptoms. Radiographically, 86% of women and 78% of men older than 65 years show evidence of osteoarthritis, but 40% to 70% of people with radiographic changes of osteoarthritis are symptom free.[6–8] Therefore, the diagnosis of osteoarthritis should be based on a combination of clinical and radiographic findings.[1]

THEORETICAL CONSIDERATIONS

Theoretical evidence regarding a proposed association between running and degenerative joint disease can be broadly classified into 3 categories: human epidemiologic evidence from non running studies, in vitro laboratory evidence, and animal studies.[1]

An association between running and the development of osteoarthritis is theoretically supported by abundant epidemiologic evidence supporting the concept that osteoarthritis is more common in joints that sustain greater loads over extended periods of time.[9–15] In addition, in vitro laboratory studies have provided evidence suggesting that the stresses of acute and repetitive joint loading can be associated with changes in articular cartilage.[16–20] In light of this evidence indicating that loading of joints in at least some form can be associated with osteoarthritis, it is reasonable to entertain the idea that repetitive loading of joints during years of running might also lead to greater wear and tear in weight-bearing joints.

GENERAL HUMAN EPIDEMIOLOGIC STUDIES

There are numerous epidemiologic studies apart from the running literature that strongly suggest an association between repetitive exposure to increased mechanical stress and the development of osteoarthritis in weight-bearing joints. Different types of abnormal loading have been identified as predisposing to osteoarthritis. These primarily include obesity, malalignment, and heavy manual labor. For a more in-depth discussion of these studies, the reader is referred elsewhere.[1,10–15,21–23] Whereas it is plausible that the results from these populations might be applicable to runners, the running-specific epidemiologic research reviewed here argues otherwise.

IN VITRO STUDIES

The ability of joints to withstand destructive forces is dependent on intrinsic and extrinsic factors. Intrinsic factors include water content, proteoglycan content, and matrix integrity of the articular cartilage; thickness of the articular cartilage; subchondral bone integrity; the ability of periarticular ligaments and muscles to support the joint; and the body's inherent healing mechanisms. Extrinsic factors include the magnitude, frequency, rate, and direction of forces applied to the joint.[1]

Several in vitro laboratory studies have provided information suggesting that joint forces in the normal physiologic range do not lead to degenerative changes. In a study of articular surface pressures, Adams and Swanson[18] used direct pressure measurements in cadaveric hip joints during simulated activity to examine the effects of physical activity on joint surfaces. The findings of this study showed that physical activities under normal conditions result in articular surface pressures ranging between 4.93 and 9.57 MN/m^2. These pressures were not observed to cause fibrillation in joint cartilage, and the investigators concluded that physiologic stresses do not cause injury to normal joints.

A related study by Repo and Finlay[24] examined survival of articular cartilage after controlled impact. Scanning electron microscopy revealed no evidence of chondrocyte death or structural damage until stress levels of 25 MN/m^2 or greater were reached. These levels of stress correlated with loads far greater than those sustained during normal physical activity.[24] The findings of this study, combined with the findings of Adams and Swanson,[18] suggest that activities such as running and jumping are not likely to result in maximal joint stresses greater than those required to cause disruption of normal articular cartilage.

In contrast to these studies suggesting that joint use within the normal physiologic range does not cause damage to articular cartilage, several in vitro studies have suggested that certain types of applied loads and repetitive motion can produce degenerative changes in joints.[1]

In one study examining the behavior of articular cartilage subjected to an applied load, Newton and colleagues[25] suggested that the ability of articular cartilage to distribute forces is dependent on the rate at which the force is applied. When a load is applied to the surface of normal articular cartilage, movement of fluid within the matrix of the cartilage occurs to optimally distribute forces throughout the cartilage and to the subchondral bone.[26] When the load is applied slowly, there is time for the fluid within the matrix to redistribute, thus allowing the cartilage to undergo appropriate deformation and absorb the impulse sustained by the macromolecular cartilaginous framework. If a force is applied too quickly for redistribution of fluid within the cartilage (eg, in sudden torsional joint loading or sudden axial joint impact during sports), a greater stress is applied to the macromolecular framework of the matrix.[26]

Examining the effects of applied loads and repetitive motion on joints, Weightman and colleagues[27] cyclically loaded in vitro samples of human cartilage to the point that fibrillation of the cartilage surface was induced. Extrapolation of the results of this study suggests that tensile fatigue failure of articular cartilage may occur at physiologic stress levels if the loads are applied at a high enough frequency.

In 3 related studies, Radin and colleagues[28–30] demonstrated articular cartilage degeneration in in vitro bovine metacarpophalangeal joints subjected to repetitive motion combined with impact loading. Their data suggested that degenerative changes may occur when in vitro articular cartilage is subjected to physiologic stress levels, if the joint is simultaneously subject to repetitive rotation in combination with axial loading.

Dekel and Weissman[31] used rabbit knee joints to investigate the effects of repetitive joint rotation versus rotation combined with axial peak overloading. The investigators in this study, as in the studies by Weightman and colleagues[27] and Radin and Paul,[28] reported physical and biochemical changes in the articular cartilage surface with these types of combined joint stress. In addition, Dekel and Weissman[31] attempted to distinguish between the 2 types of stress to which weight-bearing joints are subjected. One stress is a shear stress produced by reciprocal friction of articulating surfaces. The other is axial loading. These researchers observed degenerative changes in knees subjected to simultaneous shear stress and axial overloading, but not in those subjected to repetitive shear overuse alone. This distinction suggests that it is the added peak axial overloading that is responsible for degenerative physical and biochemical changes in joints.

Zimmerman and colleagues[32] used in vitro cartilage plugs to show that repetitive loading can be a cause of cartilage disruption. They found that the extent of damage increased as the load increased and as the number of loading cycles increased. When the investigators used 1000 psi (7×10^6 N/m^2), they found surface abrasions after 250 cycles. These observers noted primary fissures that penetrated to the calcified cartilage after 500 cycles. Secondary fissures off the primary fissures occurred after 1000 cycles, and after 8000 cycles, fissures coalesced and undercut cartilage fragments. With higher loads, similar changes were seen after fewer cycles. The findings of this study indicate that repetitive loads can cause progression of cartilage damage from surface abrasions to vertical fissures and can ultimately extend the damage to create free fragments and cartilage flaps. It must be noted, however, that the forces applied in this study are several orders of magnitude greater than those encountered under normal physiologic conditions.

An investigation of the proposed threshold of stress for joint injury by Newberry and colleagues[33] involved the impaction of rabbit patellofemoral joints at varying intensities. Their data suggest that low-intensity impacts produced acute tissue stresses lower than the injury threshold, whereas high-intensity impacts produced stresses that exceeded the threshold for disease pathogenesis.

In a general sense, these studies begin to identify safe and unsafe ranges of cartilage stress, which may have future utility in the design of safe training programs for humans. The extrapolation of these low- and high-intensity stresses from in vitro laboratory studies to human terms remains ill defined. The clinical question remains: does the act of running generate mechanical stress sufficient to cause disruption of normal articular cartilage?[1]

IN VIVO ANIMAL STUDIES

Space does not permit an exhaustive review of in vivo animal studies that have investigated the relationship between running and osteoarthritis. Taken together, the findings of these in vivo animal studies clearly indicate that running can affect the composition and mechanical properties of articular cartilage.[1] Low and moderate-volume running appear to have a beneficial effect on articular cartilage.[25,34,35] High-volume running can lead to subchondral bone changes and decreased cartilage indentation stiffness and proteoglycan concentration, but it remains unclear from these animal studies if this is equivalent to symptomatic osteoarthritis or whether it represents normal tissue adaptation.[36,37] The experimental models designed to assess the effect of running in the setting of preexisting osteoarthritis show mixed results. One study, which used a period of immobilization to induce cartilage damage, showed no worsening of osteoarthritis with running compared with control animals.[38] A second study, which used instillation of hydrogen peroxide into joints to induce cartilage damage, indicated that running does worsen osteoarthritis.[39] Finally, running too soon after an injury may lead to worse outcomes compared with resting a joint after an acute joint injury.[40,41]

HUMAN STUDIES
Studies Suggesting a Link Between Running and Osteoarthritis

There are 3 clinical reports in the human literature that suggest a link between running and osteoarthritis. The first is of dubious value because of methodological problems.

The second found an association between very high-volume running and the development of osteoarthritis. The third found an association only in a subgroup of subjects.[1]

McDermott and Freyne[9] published a report on the incidence of osteoarthritis in runners with knee pain. They evaluated 20 distance runners who complained of knee pain and found that 6 of the 20 had radiographic signs of osteoarthritis. Because 30% of the subjects had radiographic evidence of knee arthritis, the investigators suggested that distance running is a risk factor for degenerative joint disease. They appropriately cautioned, however, that there were several confounding factors. For example, the 6 runners who had radiographic evidence of knee osteoarthritis also had a higher incidence of traumatic knee injuries and greater genu varum than the 14 runners without radiographic evidence of osteoarthritis. Methodological flaws that further detract from the value of this case series include the lack of nonrunning controls, selection bias, and the omission of the cause of knee pain in most of the subjects.

In a more methodologically sound study, Marti and colleagues[42] investigated the relationship between distance running and hip osteoarthritis. They obtained histories and performed physical examinations on 27 elite distance runners, 9 bobsledders, and 23 sedentary controls. The runners had significantly more radiographic evidence of hip osteoarthritis than the bobsledders or nonrunning controls, as judged by blinded radiologists. They found age, mileage run, and running pace to be independent predictors of hip osteoarthritis. There were significantly more degenerative changes seen in the hips of those who ran an average of more than 65 mile/wk compared with those who ran less. Running pace was a stronger predictor of the development of hip osteoarthritis than running mileage. This latter finding provides clinical correlation to basic science research[25–27] that suggested that higher rates of applied load are associated with cartilage breakdown. Vo_2max was inversely correlated with radiographic findings of osteoarthritis.

Cheng and colleagues[43] reported on the relationship between self-reported physical activity and physician-diagnosed osteoarthritis from a prospective survey of nearly 17,000 patients between the ages of 20 and 87 years who were seen in their clinic between 1970 and 1995. They found no relationship between the level of physical activity and the presence of osteoarthritis in women or in men older than 50 years. However, among the subgroup of men younger than 50 years, there was an association between osteoarthritis and physical activity, including a history of running more than 20 mile/wk.

Studies Refuting a Link Between Running and Osteoarthritis

In contrast to the small volume of literature cited in the previous section, there are several published reports in the human literature that provide evidence against an association between running and the development of osteoarthritis.[1]

Panush and colleagues[44] compared runners with nonrunners to investigate a possible link between running and degenerative joint disease. They examined 17 male runners and 18 male nonrunners with a mean age of 56 years. The runners ran an average of 28 mile/wk for 12 years. The study and control groups reported no differences in pain, swelling, or other musculoskeletal complaints. There were no differences between the 2 groups in terms of musculoskeletal examinations or radiographic findings. Although the study numbers were small, the investigators concluded that their data did not support an association between running and osteoarthritis.

In a similar but larger study, Sohn and Micheli[45] retrospectively studied the effect of running on osteoarthritis of the hips and knees. They administered questionnaires to

504 former collegiate cross country runners and 287 former collegiate swimmers. The subjects ranged from 23 to 77 years of age, with a mean age of 57 years. They were between 2 and 55 years postgraduation, with a mean of 25 years postgraduation. The investigators found an incidence of severe hip or knee pain of 2% in the runners and 2.4% in the swimmers. The incidence of any knee pain was 15.5% in the runners and 19.5% in the swimmers. The incidence of surgery for osteoarthritis was 0.8% in runners and 2.1% in swimmers. No difference in joint pain was found between high-mileage (40–140 mile/wk) and low-mileage (25 mile/wk) runners. Based on these findings, Sohn and Micheli concluded that running was not associated with the development of osteoarthritis of the knees or hips.

Lane and colleagues[46] investigated long-distance running and its effect on bone density and osteoarthritis. They examined 41 runners between 50 and 72 years of age and 41 age-matched controls. Unfortunately, running distance was not recorded. They administered an extensive questionnaire, performed musculoskeletal examinations, and obtained knee radiographs on all participants. Quantitative computed tomography of the first lumbar vertebra was performed to assess bone density. The examiners were blinded to subject status. They found that the runners had a 40% greater bone density in the first lumbar vertebra in comparison to the nonrunners. There were no differences between the 2 groups with respect to abnormal radiographs, crepitus, joint stability, or clinically symptomatic osteoarthritis. These data suggest that running is not associated with osteoarthritis but does promote greater bone density.

Lane and colleagues[47] continued their investigation of the relationship between running, osteoarthritis, and bone mineral density in a subsequent study. They did a 9-year follow-up of 28 runners from 60 to 70 years of age and 27 age-matched nonrunners. They compared joint examinations, knee and hip radiographs, and quantitative computed tomography of the first lumbar vertebra. They found that the radiographic findings of osteoarthritis had progressed in both groups, but there was no significant difference in the rate of progression between the 2 groups. The runners, however, maintained a greater bone mineral density. These results strengthened their conclusions from the previous study.

Konradsen and colleagues[48] also looked at the association between long-term running and osteoarthritis. They examined 27 former competitive runners who ran 12 to 24 mile/wk for an average of 40 years and 27 age-matched sedentary controls. The mean age of both groups was 58 years. The researchers found no difference in joint alignment, range of motion, or pain. There was also no difference in the radiographic appearance of the subjects' hips, knees, or ankles. These investigators also concluded that their data did not support an association between long-term running and osteoarthritis.

In a broader study, Kohatsu and Schurman[49] looked at several risk factors for the development of knee osteoarthritis using a different perspective. Rather than comparing runners with nonrunners, these investigators performed histories, radiographs, and physical examinations on 46 subjects with severe knee osteoarthritis and 46 age-matched controls without knee osteoarthritis. They found that knee osteoarthritis was associated with higher body mass index, prior knee injury, and heavy manual labor. They found no association, however, between knee osteoarthritis and the subjects' participation in athletic activities. There were twice as many runners in the control group as in the osteoarthritis group. These data also suggest that running is not associated with the development of osteoarthritis unlike obesity, prior knee injury, and heavy manual labor.

A similar study design was used by Thelin and colleagues[50] who administered a retrospective activity survey to 825 patients with advanced knee osteoarthritis and 825 matched controls. The presence of knee arthritis was correlated with a history of participating in cutting sports, such as soccer and tennis, but there was no correlation with straight-ahead sports, such as running and cross-country skiing.

Kujala and colleagues[51] investigated knee osteoarthritis in former runners, soccer players, weight lifters, and shooters. They performed a history, physical examination, and knee radiography on 117 former world-class athletes. The examiners and radiologists were both blinded to the subjects' sport participation. Confirming prior findings, they found that knee osteoarthritis was significantly associated with prior knee injury (odds ratio 4.73) and greater body mass index (odds ratio 1.76). Radiographic evidence of osteoarthritis was seen in 31% of the weight lifters, 29% of the soccer players, 14% of the runners, and 3% of the shooters. When compared with weight lifting and soccer, running seemed to cause less osteoarthritis, although it appears to be harder on the knees than shooting.

In a cross-sectional population study, Lane and colleagues[52] looked at running and the development of musculoskeletal disability in general. The investigators compared 498 runners between 50 and 72 years of age with 365 age-matched controls. They found that the runners had less physical disability, had greater functional capacity, sought medical care less frequently, and weighed less than their nonrunning counterparts. The investigators concluded that running protected against musculoskeletal disability, although they could not comment specifically on osteoarthritis.

Ward and colleagues[53] also surveyed physical disability in runners by sending yearly questionnaires over a period of 5 to 7 years to 454 older runners (mean age, 58 years; average distance run, 25 mile/wk) and nonrunners (mean age, 62 years). They collected sociodemographic, clinical, lifestyle, and disability data. They found that 49% of the runners and 77% of the nonrunners reported some physical disability. Age, greater body mass index, strenuous work-related activity, and the use of more medications were associated with a greater likelihood of disability. In agreement with Lane and colleagues' research, their data indicate that running is not associated with increased physical disability and could even be protective against physical disability.

In a large prospective study, Hootman and colleagues[54] at the Centers for Disease Control reported on the relationship between osteoarthritis and a novel concept that they termed "physical activity joint stress." Physical activity joint stress is a measure that incorporates the frequency, duration, intensity, and specific type of physical activity. More than 5000 individuals without knee or hip osteoarthritis were surveyed. Radiographs were obtained 4, 9, and 13 years after the initial survey. Among walkers and runners, there was no association between radiographic findings of osteoarthritis and any of the individual physical activity parameters measured. Nor was any association seen between progression of osteoarthritis and the global estimate of physical activity joint stress. As with other studies, the progression of arthritic changes was positively associated with greater body mass index, older age, and a history of acute knee trauma.

Perhaps the longest longitudinal study assessing an association between running and osteoarthritis was published by Chakravarty and colleagues.[55] These researchers followed up 45 long-distance masters runners and 53 controls with serial knee radiographs over a period of 18 years. At the end of the study, there was no radiographic difference in the incidence of knee osteoarthritis between the runners and nonrunners, leading the investigators to conclude that running among older individuals is not associated with accelerated osteoarthritis.

Whereas most studies that have looked for an association between osteoarthritis and running have used plain radiography, 2 groups published prospective studies using magnetic resonance imaging (MRI) to assess the status of the articular cartilage. Wijayaratne and colleagues[56] measured the volume of the retropatellar cartilage in a group of 148 women aged 40 to –67 years over a period of 2 years. Women who self-reported a higher amount of physical activity had less reduction in the volume of the retropatellar cartilage over the study period compared with more sedentary women, suggesting that regular exercise may be beneficial for articular cartilage. In a smaller but more running-specific study, Krampla and colleagues[57] performed MRI on the knees of 7 long-distance runners at 2 points in time, 10 years apart. The same MRI machine was used with identical imaging parameters. Of the 7 runners, 6 showed no changes in their MRI findings at the 10-year follow-up point. The seventh runner showed progression of preexisting findings of arthrosis. Despite their small sample size, the researchers concluded that long-distance running does not cause osteoarthritis in otherwise normal knees.

LIMITATIONS OF EXISTING LITERATURE

The inherent limitations of the existing literature warrant discussion. One limitation is that the studies available focus on the hips and knees. There are no published studies to date on whether running might be associated with (or be protective against) degenerative changes in the ankle or lumbar spine. The existing literature also lacks more comprehensive controls. For example, the influences of running surface, athletic footwear, running gait, presence of biomechanical deficits, and cross-training have not been studied. Furthermore, many of the studies cited are primarily retrospective, although more recently there have been prospective reports as well. Prospective studies require time, patience, and careful planning because osteoarthritis usually develops over a period of many years. Another limitation is that there is scant data on the effect of running on joints that are already arthritic, although experience tells us that athletes with symptomatic disease of weight-bearing joints tend to gravitate toward lower-impact sports. Finally, and perhaps most importantly, the effect of selection bias on the existing data is unclear. For example, if a study finds that older runners have less osteoarthritis than older nonrunners, perhaps it is because individuals who previously were runners but subsequently developed osteoarthritis have already been "selected" into the nonrunning group.[1]

SUMMARY

There is strong evidence that age, prior joint injury, greater body mass index, and heavy manual labor are associated with the development of osteoarthritis. The existing literature does not support an association or causal relationship between low- or moderate-distance running and osteoarthritis.[1] The literature is inconclusive regarding a causal relationship between very-high-volume running and osteoarthritis. The study by Marti and colleagues[42] found an association between running pace and high-volume-running and osteoarthritis, whereas the study by Sohn and Micheli[45] found no difference in joint pathology between high- and low-volume runners. In general, older runners tend to be healthier than their nonrunning counterparts.

Further research is needed to investigate the following areas: the relationship between running and the development of osteoarthritis of the ankle and lumbar spine; the relationship between high-volume running and the development of osteoarthritis; the influences of running pace, surface, shoes, and gait; the utility of cartilage biomarkers[58–61] in understanding the development of osteoarthritis; and the effect of selection bias on the studies performed to date.

RECOMMENDATIONS

Patients do not generally ask, "What does the literature say?" More likely, a runner will ask, "Am I doing permanent damage to my joints? Is there anything I can do to lessen the chance of developing arthritis?" Based on the data presented, the sports medicine practitioner can feel comfortable telling patients that low- and moderate-volume running do not predispose to knee or hip osteoarthritis. The clinician might also consider making some common sense recommendations, including the use of appropriate running shoes; the use of new running shoes when indicated; running on soft surfaces; cross-training; correction of running gait abnormalities; appropriate treatment of injuries; maintenance of optimal body mass index and nutritional status; correction of biomechanical deficits; and the maximization of flexibility, strength, endurance, and motor control along the kinetic chain.[1]

ACKNOWLEDGMENTS

The authors would like to thank Charis Wren for her assistance with the preparation of this manuscript.

REFERENCES

1. Willick S. Running and osteoarthritis. In: O'Connor F, Wilder R, editors. Textbook of running medicine. New York: McGraw-Hill; 2001. p. 387–94.
2. Powell KE, Paffenbarger RS. Workshop on epidemiologic and public health aspects of physical activity and exercise: a summary. Public Health Rep 1985; 100:118–26.
3. Sherwood DE, Selder DJ. Cardiorespiratory health, reaction time, and aging. Med Sci Sports 1979;11(2):186–9.
4. Buckwalter JA. Osteoarthritis and articular cartilage use, disuse, and abuse: experimental studies. J Rheumatol Suppl 1995;43:13–5.
5. Lane NE, Buckwalter JA. Exercise: a cause of osteoarthritis? Rheum Dis Clin North Am 1993;19:617–33.
6. Alexander CJ. Osteoarthritis: a review of old myths and current concepts. Skeletal Radiol 1990;19:327–33.
7. Lane NE, Michel B, Bjorkengren A, et al. The risk of osteoarthritis with running and aging. J Rheumatol 1993;20:661–8.
8. Panush RS, Lane NE. Exercise and the musculoskeletal system. Baillieres Clin Rheumatol 1994;8(1):79–103.
9. McDermott M, Freyne P. Osteoarthritis in runners with knee pain. Br J Sports Med 1983;17:84–7.
10. Lindberg H, Montgomery F. Heavy labor and the occurrence of arthrosis. Clin Orthop 1987;214:235–6.
11. Davis MA, Ettinger WH, Neuhaus JM, et al. The association of knee injury and obesity with bilateral osteoarthritis of the knee. Am J Epidemiol 1989;130(2): 278–88.
12. Felson DT, Hannan MT, Naimark A, et al. Occupational physical demands, knee bending, and knee osteoarthritis: results from the Framingham study. J Rheumatol 1991;18:1587–92.
13. Felson DT, Zhang Y, Anthony JM, et al. Weight loss reduces the risk for symptomatic knee osteoarthritis in women. The Framingham study. Ann Intern Med 1992; 116(7):535–9.
14. Paty JG. Running injuries. Curr Opin Rheumatol 1994;2:203–9.

15. Buckwalter JA, Mankin HJ. Articular cartilage: degeneration and osteoarthritis, repair, regeneration, and transplantation. Instr Course Lect 1998;47:487–503.
16. Brown TD, Shaw DT. In vitro contact stress distributions in the natural human hip. J Biomech 1983;16:373–84.
17. Miyanaga Y, Fukubayashi T, Kurosawa H. Contact study of the hip joint: Load deformation pattern, contact area and contact pressure. Arch Orthop Trauma Surg 1984;103:13–7.
18. Adams D, Swanson SA. Direct measurement of local pressures in the cadaveric human hip joint during simulated level walking. Ann Rheum Dis 1985;44:658–66.
19. Brown TD, Anderson DD, Nepola JV, et al. Contact stress aberrations following imprecise reduction of simple tibial plateau fractures. J Orthop Res 1988;6:851–62.
20. Brown TD, Pope DF, Hale JE, et al. Effects of osteochondral defect size on cartilage contact stress. J Orthop Res 1991;9:559–67.
21. Yoshimura N, Nishioka S, Kinoshita H, et al. Risk factors for knee osteoarthritis in Japanese women: heavy weight, previous joint injuries, and occupational activities. J Rheumatol 2004;31(1):157–62.
22. Yoshimura N, Kinoshita H, Hori N, et al. Risk factors for knee osteoarthritis in Japanese men: a case-control study. Mod Rheumatol 2006;16(1):24–9.
23. Seidler A, Bolm-Audorff U, Abolmaali N, et al. The role of cumulative physical work load in symptomatic knee osteoarthritis-a case-control study in Germany. J Occup Med Toxicol 2008;3(1):14.
24. Repo RU, Finlay JB. Survival of articular cartilage after controlled impact. J Bone Joint Surg Am 1977;59:1068–76.
25. Newton PM, Mow VC, Gardner TR, et al. The effect of lifelong exercise on canine articular cartilage. Am J Sports Med 1997;25:282–7.
26. Mow V, Rosenwasser M. Articular cartilage: biomechanics. In: Woo SL, Buckwalter JA, editors, Injury and repair of the musculoskeletal soft tissues, vol. 1. Park Ridge (IL): American Academy of Orthopedic Surgeons; 1988. p. 427–63.
27. Weightman B, Chappell DJ, Jenkins EA. A second study of tensile fatigue properties of human cartilage. Ann Rheum Dis 1978;37(1):58–63.
28. Radin EL, Paul IL. Response of joints to impact loading: in vitro wear. Arthritis Rheum 1971;14:356–62.
29. Radin EL, Ehrlich MG, Chemack R, et al. Effect of repetitive impulse loading on the knee joint of rabbits. Clin Orthop 1978;131:288–93.
30. Radin EL, Martin RB, Burr DB, et al. Effects of mechanical loading on the tissues of rabbit knee. J Orthop Res 1984;2:221–34.
31. Dekel S, Weissman SL. Joint changes after overuse and peak overloading of rabbit knees in vivo. Acta Orthop Scand 1978;49:519–28.
32. Zimmerman NB, Smith DG, Pottenger LA, et al. Mechanical disruption of human patellar cartilage by repetitive loading in vitro. Clin Orthop 1988;229:302–7.
33. Newberry WN, Garcia JJ, Mackenzie CD, et al. Analysis of acute mechanical stress in an animal model of post-traumatic osteoarthritis. J Biomech Eng 1998;120(6):704–9.
34. Kiviranta I, Tammi M, Jurvelin J, et al. Moderate running exercise augments glycosaminoglycans and thickness of articular cartilage in the knee joint of young beagle dogs. J Orthop Res 1988;16:188–95.
35. Kiviranta I, Tammi M, Jurvelin J, et al. Articular cartilage thickness and glycosaminoglycan distribution in the canine knee joint after strenuous running exercise. Clin Orthop 1992;283:302–8.

36. Oettmeier R, Arokoski J, Roth AJ, et al. Subchondral bone and articular cartilage response to long distance running training (40 km per day) in the beagle knee joint. Eur J Exp Musculoskel Res 1992;1:145–54.

37. Arokoski J, Kiviranta I, Jurvelin J, et al. Long-distance running causes site-dependent decrease of cartilage glycosaminoglycan content in the knee joints of beagle dogs. Arthritis Rheum 1993;36:1451–9.

38. Videman T. The effect of running on the osteoarthritic joint: an experimental matched-pair study with rabbits. Rheumatol Rehabil 1982;21:1–8.

39. Kaiki G, Suji H, Yonesawa T, et al. Osteoarthritis induced by intra-articular hydrogen peroxide injection and running load. J Orthop Res 1990;8:730–40.

40. Palmoski MJ, Brandt KD. Running inhibits the reversal of atrophic changes in canine knee cartilage after removal of a leg cast. Arthritis Rheum 1981;24: 1329–37.

41. Palmoski MJ, Brandt KD. Immobilization of the knee prevents osteoarthritis after anterior cruciate ligament resection. Arthritis Rheum 1982;25:1201–8.

42. Marti B, Knobloch M, Tschopp A, et al. Is excessive running predictive of degenerative hip disease? Br Med J 1989;299:91–3.

43. Cheng Y, Macera CA, Davis DR, et al. Physical activity and self-reported, physician-diagnosed osteoarthritis: is physical activity a risk factor? J Clin Epidemiol 2000;53(3):315–22.

44. Panush RS, Schmidt C, Caldwell JR, et al. Is running associated with degenerative joint disease? JAMA 1986;255(14):1152–4.

45. Sohn RS, Micheli LJ. The effect of running on the pathogenesis of osteoarthritis of the hips and knees. Clin Orthop Relat Res 1985;198:106–9.

46. Lane NE, Bloch DA, Jones HH, et al. Long-distance running, bone density, and osteoarthritis. JAMA 1986;255:1141–51.

47. Lane NE, Oehlert JW, Bloch DA, et al. The relationship of running to osteoarthritis of the knee and hip and bone mineral density of the lumbar spine: a 9 year longitudinal study. J Rheumatol 1998;25:334–41.

48. Konradsen L, Hansen EM, Songard L. Long distance running and osteoarthritis. Am J Sports Med 1990;18:379–81.

49. Kohatsu ND, Schurman DJ. Risk factors for the development of osteoarthritis of the knee. Clin Orthop Relat Res 1990;261:242–6.

50. Thelin N, Holmberg S, Thelin A. Knee injuries account for the sports-related increased risk of knee osteoarthritis. Scand J Med Sci Sports 2006;16(5): 329–33.

51. Kujala UM, Kettunen J, Paananen H, et al. Knee osteoarthritis in former runners, soccer players, weight lifters, and shooters. Arthritis Rheum 1995;38:539–46.

52. Lane NE, Bloch DA, Wood PD, et al. Aging, long-distance running, and the development of musculoskeletal disability. Am J Med 1987;82:772–80.

53. Ward MM, Hubert HB, Shi H, et al. Physical disability in older runners: prevalence, risk factors, and progression with age. J Gerontol A Biol Sci Med Sci 1995;50:M70–7.

54. Hootman JM, Macera CA, Helmick CG, et al. Influence of physical activity-related joint stress on the risk of self-reported hip/knee osteoarthritis: a new method to quantify physical activity. Prev Med 2003;36(5):636–44.

55. Chakravarty EF, Hubert HB, Lingala VB, et al. Long distance running and knee osteoarthritis. A prospective study. Am J Prev Med 2008;35(2):133–8.

56. Wijayaratne SP, Teichtahl AJ, Wluka AE, et al. The determinants of change in patella cartilage volume—a cohort study of healthy middle-aged women. Rheumatology 2008;47(9):1426–9.

57. Krampla WW, Newrkla SP, Kroener AH, et al. Changes on magnetic resonance tomography in the knee joints of marathon runners: a 10-year longitudinal study. Skeletal Radiol 2008;37(7):619–26.

58. Neidhart M, Muller-Ladner U, Frey W, et al. Increased serum levels of non-collagenous matrix proteins (cartilage oligomeric matrix protein and melanoma inhibitory activity) in marathon runners. Osteoarthr Cartil 2000;8(3):222–9.

59. Kersting UG, Stubendorff JJ, Schmidt MC, et al. Changes in knee cartilage volume and serum COMP concentration after running exercise. Osteoarthr Cartil 2005;13(10):925–34.

60. O'Kane JW, Hutchinson E, Atley LM, et al. Sport-related differences in biomarkers of bone resorption and cartilage degradation in edurance athletes. Osteoarthr Cartil 2006;14(1):71–6.

61. Kim HJ, Lee YH, Kim CK. Biomarkers of muscle and cartilage damage and inflammation during a 200 km run. Eur J Appl Physiol 2007;99(4):443–7.

Exertional Compartment Syndrome

Robert P. Wilder, MD[a],*, Eric Magrum, PT[b]

KEYWORDS
- Exertional compartment syndrome • Running injury
- Pressure monitoring • Fasciotomy

Chronic exertional compartment syndrome is defined as reversible ischemia secondary to a noncompliant osseofascial compartment that is unresponsive to the expansion of muscle volume that occurs with exercise.[1,2] Most commonly seen in the lower leg, exertional compartment syndrome in athletes has also been described in the thigh and medial compartment of the foot.[3–5] The syndrome presents as recurrent episodes of leg discomfort experienced at a given distance or intensity of running. Although a characteristic history is highly suggestive of exertional compartment syndrome, no physical examination finding can firmly establish the diagnosis.[2,6,7] Diagnosis based solely on clinical presentation can lead to misdiagnosis and inappropriate therapy or delay of proper therapy.[8] An exercise challenge and documentation of elevated compartment pressure in one or more of the compartments of the leg confirms the diagnosis.[1,2]

The characteristic presenting complaint of patients with chronic exertional compartment syndrome is recurrent exercise-induced leg discomfort that occurs at a well-defined and reproducible point in the run and increases if the training persists. The quality of pain is usually described as a tight, cramplike, or squeezing ache over a specific compartment of the leg. Athletes can reliably predict at what intensity or what distances the discomfort will occur as well as how long pain will last, depending on the intensity and distance run. Relief of symptoms only occurs with discontinuation of activity.[9] Examination may or may not demonstrate fascial hernias. In some cases, the classic exertional component is not as evident, and patients complain of pain at rest or with daily activities as well. Women may be more susceptible to chronic lower leg compartment syndrome than men, and women may also, for unclear reasons,

---

[a] Department of PM&R, University of Virginia, 545 Ray C. Hunt #240, Charlottesville, VA 22901, USA
[b] UVa Health South Physical Therapy, 545 Ray C. Hunt, Suite 240, Charlottesville, VA, USA
* Corresponding author.
E-mail address: rpw4n@virginia.edu

Clin Sports Med 29 (2010) 429–435
doi:10.1016/j.csm.2010.03.008
0278-5919/10/$ – see front matter © 2010 Published by Elsevier Inc.

sportsmed.theclinics.com

respond less well than men to operative fasciotomy.[10] Chronic compartment syndrome, left untreated, can develop into an acute syndrome.[11]

The differential diagnosis of chronic exertional compartment syndrome is listed in **Box 1**.[7] Clinicians should be aware that more than one contributor may be present. In an unpublished review of more than 100 athletes with compartment syndrome seen at the Runner's Clinic at the University of Virginia, nearly 30% also had a stress fracture of the tibia or fibula.

Several factors are thought to contribute to an increase in intracompartmental pressure during exercise[1,7,9,12]: enclosure of compartmental contents in an inelastic fascial sheath, increased volume of the skeletal muscle with exertion due to blood flow and edema, dynamic contraction factors due to the gait cycle, and muscle hypertrophy as a response to exercise. It has also been proposed that myofiber damage as a result of eccentric exercise causes a release of protein-bound ions and a subsequent increase in osmotic pressure within the compartment. The increase in osmotic pressure increases capillary relaxation pressure, thus decreasing the blood flow.[13] Development of symptoms may be more common at the beginning of a running season due to muscle hypertrophy, which decreases the volume in the compartment.[14] Rapid increases in muscle size due to fluid retention are also thought to play a role in the development of chronic exertional compartment syndrome in athletes taking the popular supplement creatine.[9]

A neurologic and vascular examination should be performed with reproduction of the symptoms.[2] Understanding the distribution of nerves and functions of muscles in relation to symptoms can help identify the affected compartment in cases where the pain is not well localized to one specific compartment, or it may help determine which compartments are more severely affected in cases where more than one compartment is involved.[1,7,9]

There are 4 major compartments in the leg. Each is bound by bone and fascia, and each contains a major nerve. The anterior compartment contains the extensor hallucis

---

Box 1
Differential diagnosis of exertional leg pain

Chronic exertional compartment syndrome

Medial tibial stress syndrome

Stress fracture

Tenosynovitis

Periostitis

Deep venous thrombosis

Nerve entrapment syndrome

Lumbosacral radiculopathy

Neurogenic Claudication

Popliteal artery entrapment syndrome

Vascular claudication

Infection

Myopathy

Tumor

longus, extensor digitorum longus, peroneus tertius, and anterior tibialis muscles, as well as the deep peroneal nerve. The lateral compartment contains the peroneus longus and brevis as well as the superficial peroneal nerve. Posteriorly there are 2 compartments, the superficial posterior and the deep posterior compartments. The superficial compartment contains the gastrocnemius and soleus muscles and the sural nerve. The deep posterior compartment contains the flexor hallucis longus, flexor digitorum longus, and posterior tibialis muscles, and the posterior tibial nerve. Some investigators believe that the posterior tibialis should be considered a separate compartment because it is surrounded by its own fascia.[1,15] Anterior compartment syndrome is most common (45%), followed by the deep posterior compartment (40%), lateral compartment (10%), and superficial posterior compartments (5%).[13]

If the anterior compartment is affected, the patient may display weakness of dorsiflexion or toe extension and paresthesias over the dorsum of the foot, numbness in the first web space, or even transient or persistent foot drop.[2,14] Paresthesias in the plantar aspect of the foot and weakness of toe flexion and foot inversion may be revealed when the deep posterior compartment is involved, whereas dorsolateral foot hypoesthesia and plantar flexion weakness may be present if the superficial posterior compartment is affected. Lateral compartment pressure elevation with compression of the superficial peroneal nerve can induce sensory changes over the anterolateral aspect of the leg and weakness of ankle eversion. An inversion as well as equinus deformity may also be present.[2,16]

Several techniques have been described in the literature for measuring both static and dynamic intramuscular pressures.[1] These techniques include the needle manometer,[17] wick catheter,[18] slit catheter,[19] continuous infusion,[20] and solid-state transducer intracompartmental catheter.[21] Each of these techniques offers several advantages and disadvantages. However, all are time consuming and require some degree of skill and experience to set up and perform.[2,9]

The authors' preferred method for measurement of compartmental pressures is with a battery-operated, hand-held, digital, fluid pressure monitor. The Stryker Intracompartmental Pressure Monitor (Stryker Corp, Kalamazoo, MI, USA) is a convenient and easy-to-use measuring device for use in the clinical setting.[1,2,21] This device has been found to be more accurate, versatile, convenient, and much less time consuming to use than the needle manometer method.[22] Measurements were also found to be more reproducible among different examiners with the Stryker instrument.[2]

The usefulness of pressure measurement and maintenance of patient safety with this invasive technique relies on a thorough knowledge of the anatomy of the leg. Before attempting to measure compartment pressures, the physician should thoroughly study the anatomic structures in each compartment to avoid damaging neurovascular structures.[2]

Generally accepted criteria for the diagnosis of chronic exertional compartment syndrome are described by Pedowitz and colleagues.[8] One or more of the following pressure criteria must be met in addition to a history and physical examination that is consistent with the diagnosis of chronic exertional compartment syndrome; the greater number of criteria satisfied, the greater level of confidence in the diagnosis[7]: preexercise pressure 15 mm Hg or greater; 1 minute postexercise pressure 30 mm Hg or greater; or 5 minutes postexercise pressure 20 mm Hg or greater. In patients with chronic exertional compartment syndrome, pressures may remain elevated for 30 minutes or longer.[7] Clinicians should also be aware that standard exercise protocols often used in the clinical setting may or may not be adequate to raise intracompartmental pressure, and diagnosis may require the sport-specific activity to induce symptoms and raise intracompartmental pressure.[23]

Recent interest has focused on the use of noninvasive tools in the diagnosis of chronic compartment syndrome: triple-phase bone scan, magnetic resonance imaging (MRI), near-infrared spectroscopy, methoxyisobutyl isonitrile (MIBI) perfusion imaging, and thallous chloride scintigraphy.[1,7,24–33]

The dynamic bone scan may support the diagnosis based on specific tracer uptake patterns. The characteristic appearance is that of decreased radionuclide concentration in the vicinity of the area of increased pressure, with increased soft tissue concentration both superior and inferior to the abnormality. The area of decreased uptake is thought to be caused by the increased pressure and decreased blood flow to the region.[28] On MRI, exercise changes are characterized by swelling within a compartment, which manifests as intramuscular diffuse high signal intensity on T2-weighted images. Failure of the edematous muscle to return to normal baseline appearance by 25 minutes after completion of exercise is diagnostic.[29] The triple-phase bone scan and MRI offer alternatives to direct intracompartmental pressure measurements in cases where the athlete is adverse to repeated needle sticks or when the results of pressure monitoring may be borderline.[2,30]

Near-infrared spectroscopy measures tissue deoxygenation of skeletal muscle caused by elevated intramuscular pressure during exercise.[25] Thallous chloride scintigraphy with single-photon emission computed tomography scanning was reported to demonstrate reversible ischemia in affected compartments during exercise.[7,33]

MIBI perfusion imaging is a technique that assesses the uptake of an intravenously injected radiopharmaceutical, technetium-99m MIBI, by peripheral muscles. The uptake of the radiopharmaceutical is largely determined by muscle perfusion but hypoxia also inhibits uptake of the MIBI, enhancing its potential for detecting muscle ischemia. Cases have been reported in which visually detectable decreases in MIBI uptake in one or more compartments were noted during exercise when compared with measurements taken at rest.[26]

Treatment of chronic exertional compartment syndrome can include both conservative and surgical intervention.[1] Conservative measures include relative rest (limiting activity to that level which avoids any more than minimal symptoms), anti-inflammatories, manual therapy and soft tissue release, stretching and strengthening of the involved muscles, and orthotics (particularly in cases of excessive pronation). Some athletes will simply choose to refrain from the causative activity, which is a viable option provided they remain neurovascularly intact.

Should symptoms persist despite 6 to 12 weeks of conservative care, or in cases of extreme pressure elevation, surgical remediation (fasciotomy of the involved compartments with or without fasciectomy) should be undertaken.[34–39] Single and double incision as well as endoscopic techniques have been described. Regardless of the technique, any fascial hernias must be included in the fascial incision. Surgical treatment generally has good success with return to running, without significant symptoms. Anterior compartment fasciotomy success rates usually exceed 85%. Deep posterior success rates are lower, approximately 70%.[7]

Due to a high rate of coexistence, some investigators advocate release of the lateral compartment whenever a procedure for anterior compartment syndrome is performed. Others have stated that this dual release may not be necessary if clinical evaluation and compartment pressure testing fail to demonstrate lateral compartment involvement.[40] When performing a deep posterior compartment release, attention must be given to adequate decompression of the tibialis posterior.[41]

A compressive dressing is applied postoperatively. Drains are not normally necessary. Crutches are used for comfort for a few days, but the patient begins active and passive motion immediately. Once the wound is healed, walking and cycling are encouraged. Patients may begin a light jog in 2 weeks, and resume run training at 6 weeks. Full rehabilitation usually takes 3 months, but patients with deep posterior compartment fasciotomies may need longer.[7,15,42]

REFERENCES

1. Wilder RP, Sethi S. Overuse injuries; tendinopathies, stress fractures, compartment syndrome and shin splints. Clin Sports Med 2004;23:55–81.
2. Glorioso J, Wilckens J. Compartment syndrome testing. In: O'Connor F, Wilder R, editors. The textbook of running medicine. New York: McGraw-Hill; 2001. p. 95–100.
3. Raether PM, Lutter LD. Recurrent compartment syndrome in the posterior thigh. Report of a case. Am J Sports Med 1982;10(1):40–3.
4. Birnbaum J. Recurrent compartment syndrome in the posterior thigh. Am J Sports Med 1983;11(1):48–9.
5. Mollica MB, Duyshart SC. Analysis of pre- and post-exercise compartment pressures in the medial compartment of the foot. Am J Sports Med 2002;30(2):268–71.
6. Styf JR, Korner LM. Diagnosis of chronic anterior compartment syndrome in the lower leg. Acta Orthop Scand 1987;58(2):139–44.
7. Rowden GA, Abdelkarim B, Vaca F. Compartment syndromes. eMedicine from WebMD, Medscape, October 29, 2008. [Online].
8. Pedowitz RA, Hargens AR, Mubarak SJ, et al. Modified criteria for the objective diagnosis of chronic compartment syndrome of the leg. Am J Sports Med 1990;18(1):35–40.
9. Glorioso J, Wilckens J. Exertional leg pain. In: O'Connor F, Wilder R, editors. The textbook of running medicine. New York: McGraw-Hill; 2001. p. 181–98.
10. Micheli LJ, Solomon R, Solomon J, et al. Surgical treatment for chronic lower-leg compartment syndrome in young female athletes. Am J Sports Med 1999;27(2): 197–201.
11. Mubarak SJ, Owen CA, Garfin S, et al. Acute exertional superficial posterior compartment syndrome. Am J Sports Med 1978;6(5):287–90.
12. McDermott AG, Marble AE, Yabsley RH, et al. Monitoring dynamic anterior compartment pressures during exercise. A new technique using the STIC catheter. Am J Sports Med 1982;10(2):83–9.
13. Edwards P, Myerson M. Exertional compartment syndrome of the leg: steps for expedient return to activity. Phys Sportsmed 1996;24:31–46.
14. Detmer DE, Sharpe K, Sufit RI, et al. Chronic compartment syndrome: diagnosis, management, and outcomes. Am J Sports Med 1985;13(3):162–70.
15. Albertson K, Dammann G. The leg. In: O'Connor F, Wilder R, editors. The textbook of running medicine. New York: McGraw-Hill; 2001. p. 647–54.
16. Gordon G. Leg pains in athletes. J Foot Surg 1979;18(2):55–8.
17. Whitesides TE Jr, Haney TC, Harada H, et al. A simple method for tissue pressure determination. Arch Surg 1975;110(11):1311–3.
18. Mubarak SJ, Hargens AR, Owen CA, et al. The wick catheter technique for measurement of intramuscular pressure. A new research and clinical tool. J Bone Joint Surg Am 1976;58(7):1016–20.
19. Rorabeck CH, Castle GS, Hardie R, et al. Compartmental pressure measurements: an experimental investigation using the slit catheter. J Trauma 1981; 21(6):446–9.
20. Matsen FA 3rd, Mayo KA, Sheridan GW, et al. Monitoring of intramuscular pressure. Surgery 1976;79(6):702–9.

21. Hutchinson M, Ireland M. Chronic exertional compartment syndrome—gauging pressure. Phys Sportsmed 1999;27:101.

22. Awbrey BJ, Sienkiewicz PS, Mankin HJ. Chronic exercise-induced compartment pressure elevation measured with a miniaturized fluid pressure monitor. A laboratory and clinical study. Am J Sports Med 1988;16(6):610–5.

23. Padhiar N, King JB. Exercise induced leg pain-chronic compartment syndrome. Is the increase in intra-compartment pressure exercise specific? Br J Sports Med 1996;30(4):360–2.

24. Jimenez C, Allen T, Hwang I. Diagnostic imaging of running injuries. In: O'Connor F, Wilder R, editors. The textbook of running medicine. New York: McGraw-Hill; 2001. p. 67–84.

25. Breit GA, Gross JH, Watenpaugh DE. Near-infrared spectroscopy for monitoring of tissue oxygenation of exercising skeletal muscle in a chronic compartment syndrome model. J Bone Joint Surg Am 1997;79:838–43.

26. Owens S, Edwards P, Miles K, et al. Chronic compartment syndrome affecting the lower limb: MIBI perfusion imaging as an alternative to pressure monitoring: two case reports. Br J Sports Med 1999;33(1):49–51.

27. Samuelson DR, Cram RL. The three-phase bone scan and exercise induced lower-leg pain. The tibial stress test. Clin Nucl Med 1996;21(2):89–93.

28. Matin P. Basic principles of nuclear medicine techniques for detection and evaluation of trauma and sports medicine injuries. Semin Nucl Med 1988;18(2): 90–112.

29. Kaplan P, Helms C, Dussault R. Musculoskeletal MRI. Philadelphia: W.B. Saunders; 2001.

30. Amendola A, Rorabeck CH, Vellett D, et al. The use of magnetic resonance imaging in exertional compartment syndromes. Am J Sports Med 1990;18(1): 29–34.

31. Eskelin MK, Lotjonen JM, Mantysaari MJ. Chronic exertional compartment syndrome: MR imaging at 0.1 T compared with tissue pressure measurement. [comment]. Radiology 1998;206(2):333–7.

32. Mattila KT, Komu ME, Dahlstrom S, et al. Medial tibial pain: a dynamic contrast-enhanced MRI study. Magn Reson Imaging 1999;17(7):947–54.

33. Hayes AA, Bower GD, Pitstock KL. Chronic exertional compartment syndrome of the legs diagnosed with thallous chloride scintigraphy. J Nucl Med 1995;36: 1618–24.

34. Leversedge FJ, Casey PJ, Seiler JG 3rd, et al. Endoscopically assisted fasciotomy: description of technique and in vitro assessment of lower-leg compartment decompression. Am J Sports Med 2002;30(2):272–8.

35. Slimmon D, Bennell K, Brukner P, et al. Long-term outcome of fasciotomy with partial fasciectomy for chronic exertional compartment syndrome of the lower leg. Am J Sports Med 2002;30(4):581–8.

36. Raikin SM, Rapuri VR, Vitanzo P. Bilateral simultaneous fasciotomy for chronic exertional compartment syndrome. Foot Ankle Int 2005;26:1007–11.

37. Mouhsine E, Gorofalo R, Moretti B, et al. Two minimal incision fasciotomy for chronic exertional compartment syndrome of the lower leg. Knee Surg Sports Traumatol Arthrosc 2006;14:193–7.

38. Tzortziou V, Maffulli N, Padhiar N. Diagnosis and management of chronic exertional compartment syndrome (CECS) in the United Kingdom. Clin J Sport Med 2006;16:209–13.

39. Wittstein J, Moorman CT, Levin LS. Endoscopic compartment release for chronic exertional compartment syndrome. J Surg Orthop Adv 2008;17:119–21.

40. Schepsis AA, Gill SS, Foster TA. Fasciotomy for exertional anterior compartment syndrome: is lateral compartment release necessary? Am J Sports Med 1999; 27(4):430–5.
41. Davey JR, Rorabeck CH, Fowler PJ. The tibialis posterior muscle compartment. An unrecognized cause of exertional compartment syndrome. Am J Sports Med 1984;12(5):391–7.
42. Rorabeck CH. The diagnosis and management of chronic compartment syndromes. Instr Course Lect 1989;38:466.

Neuropathies in Runners

Evan Peck, MD, Jonathan T. Finnoff, DO, Jay Smith, MD*

KEYWORDS

- Neuropathy • Sports • Running • Athletes

Nerve entrapment is an uncommon source of lower limb pain in runners, but has received increasing attention since Massey and colleagues[1] published a report of peroneal (PN) and lateral femoral cutaneous (LFCN) neuropathies in runners. Neurologic conditions currently account for 10% to 15% of all exercise-induced leg pain among runners, representing the highest frequency of foot and ankle neurologic conditions among all athletes.[2–5] Most nerve entrapments occur secondary to nonpenetrating trauma. Specific causes include contusion, compression, stretch, and iatrogenic injury from surgery.[2,5–10] The running motion produces complex, forceful, and repetitive lower limb movements that may compress, stretch, or dislocate nerves as they traverse relatively unyielding musculotendinous or fibro-osseous compartments and tunnels. Repetitive trauma produces demyelination (neuropraxia), and potentially some degree of axonal loss (axonotmesis); nerve dysfunction and neuropathic pain ensues.[11] Neurotmesis (complete nerve transection) does not occur in runners without major trauma.

In order of decreasing frequency, the most common nerves affected in runners include the interdigital nerve (interdigital or Morton neuroma), first branch of the lateral plantar nerve (FB-LPN), medial plantar nerve (MPN), tibial nerve (TN), peroneal nerve (common [CPN], as well as deep [DPN] and superficial [SPN]), sural nerve (SN), and saphenous nerve.[5] This article reviews the causes, diagnosis, and treatment of entrapment neuropathies that may be encountered by clinicians caring for runners.

DIAGNOSTIC PRINCIPLES

Clinicians should consider several general principles to facilitate the diagnosis and management of entrapment neuropathies: (1) maintain a high index of suspicion for neurologic syndromes, (2) recognize common presentations of neuropathic pain, (3) perform a meticulous physical examination, including postexercise examination when necessary, (4) consider a broad differential diagnosis (neurologic and nonneurologic), (5) use diagnostic testing appropriately, and (6) make rational clinical decisions,

Department of Physical Medicine and Rehabilitation, Mayo Clinic Sports Medicine Center, Mayo Clinic, 200 First Street SW, Rochester, MN 55905, USA
* Corresponding author.
E-mail address: smith.jay@mayo.edu

Clin Sports Med 29 (2010) 437–457
doi:10.1016/j.csm.2010.03.002
0278-5919/10/$ – see front matter © 2010 Elsevier Inc. All rights reserved.

sportsmed.theclinics.com

including referral for second opinion when indicated.[5] **Figs. 1–7** depict the relevant neuroanatomy as it pertains to entrapment or injury sites. **Fig 8** presents the neuroanatomic relationship of nerves in the lower limb.

COMMON NERVE ENTRAPMENT SYNDROMES
Interdigital Neuroma (Morton Neuroma)

Definition
Interdigital neuromas produce neuropathic pain in the distribution of the interdigital nerve (see **Fig. 1**). The condition most commonly affects the third web space, and rarely affects the first or fourth web spaces. Multiple coexistent neuromas are uncommon and suggest an alternative diagnosis such as polyneuropathy. Interdigital neuromas typically affect runners in their 20s or older, show a predilection for women (possibly secondary to wearing tight-fitting and high-heeled dress shoes), and are believed to be caused by repetitive trauma and biomechanical factors.[2,5,7,10,12]

Anatomy, pathophysiology, and risk factors
The plantar interdigital nerve in the third intermetatarsal space is comprised of communicating branches from the LPN and MPN (see **Figs. 8** and **2**). At the level of the metatarsal heads, the interdigital nerve passes plantar to the intermetatarsal ligament. During push-off, forceful toe dorsiflexion may compress and stretch the nerve beneath the intermetatarsal ligament, resulting in demyelination, scarring, and hypertrophy.[2,10] Subsequently, a tumorous mass may develop just distal to the intermetatarsal ligament, proximal to the interdigital nerve's bifurcation into the deep digital

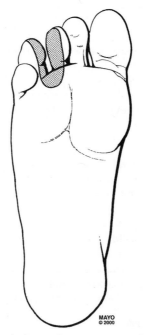

Fig. 1. Interdigital neuroma. Shaded area demonstrates typical area of pain or sensory loss. (By permission of Mayo Foundation for Medical Education and Research. All rights reserved.)

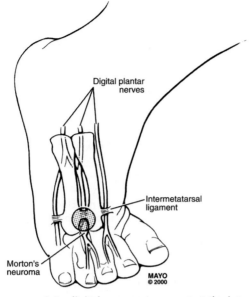

Fig. 2. Interdigital neuroma. Interdigital nerve entrapment at the intermetatarsal ligament. (By permission of Mayo Foundation for Medical Education and Research. All rights reserved.)

plantar nerves. Histologically, there is typically prominent perineural and endoneural fibrosis, with a lesser degree of demyelination.[7]

General risk factors include prolonged walking or running (especially during push-off), squatting, use of high-heeled or narrow toe-boxed shoes, or the demi-pointe in ballet.[2,12] In runners, several contributing conditions may coexist. Hyperpronation dorsiflexes the third metatarsal relative to the fourth, exposing the nerve to injury during push-off.[5] Hallux valgus or a hypermobile first ray may lead to callous formation on the plantar aspects of the metatarsal heads, increasing intermetatarsal pressures.

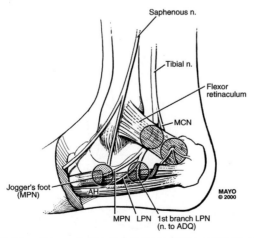

Fig. 3. Tibial nerve and tarsal tunnel. Shaded areas indicate common entrapment sites. (By permission of Mayo Foundation for Medical Education and Research. All rights reserved.)

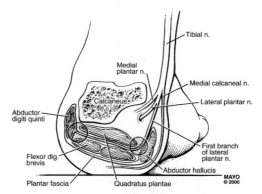

Fig. 4. First branch of lateral plantar nerve (FB-LPN). The FB-LPN courses laterally between the flexor digitorum brevis and quadratus plantae muscles. Shaded areas indicate entrapment sites. (By permission of Mayo Foundation for Medical Education and Research. All rights reserved.)

Idiopathic metatarsophalangeal joint (MTJ) synovitis may cause local edema and interdigital nerve compression.[7] Softer-soled footwear or a heel lift may precipitate symptoms as a result of increased toe dorsiflexion.

Symptoms and signs
The athlete describes neuropathic pain radiating between the third and fourth toes that is increased with running, standing, walking, toe dorsiflexion, and squatting. Burning

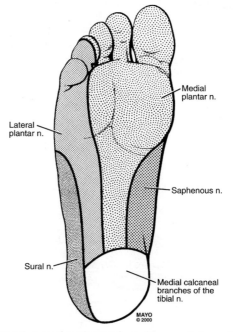

Fig. 5. Cutaneous innervation to the plantar foot. (By permission of Mayo Foundation for Medical Education and Research. All rights reserved.)

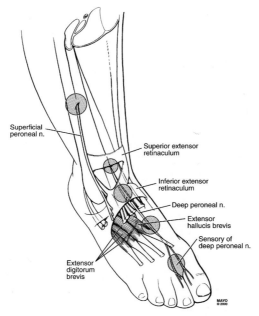

Superficial peroneal n.

Superior extensor retinaculum

Inferior extensor retinaculum

Deep peroneal n.

Extensor hallucis brevis

Sensory of deep peroneal n.

Extensor digitorum brevis

Fig. 6. Superficial and deep peroneal nerves: Shaded areas represent potential entrapment sites. (By permission of Mayo Foundation for Medical Education and Research. All rights reserved.)

and cramping are common; night pain has been reported. Relieving measures include footwear removal and massaging the forefoot.

Examination focuses on biomechanical assessment and provocative testing. The athlete is often tender in the affected intermetatarsal space. Provocative testing includes pressure application over the plantar aspect of the web space between the metatarsal heads, or squeezing the metatarsals together during palpation (metatarsal squeeze test); distal radiating neuropathic pain suggests the diagnosis. The squeeze test may also result in a click as the neuroma subluxes from between the metatarsals in a plantar direction (Mulder click).[5] A web space sensory deficit is occasionally seen, but no motor deficit is expected to occur along the purely sensory nerve. Palpation and motion testing of the MTJs may reveal subluxations or synovitis. Predisposing biomechanical factors should be determined.[2]

Differential diagnosis and evaluation
Proximal tenderness or tenderness in all of the intermetatarsal spaces should alert the clinician to consider alternative diagnoses. Differential diagnosis includes proximal and systemic neurologic conditions; stress fractures; MTJ synovitis, instability, or arthritis; and flexor-extensor tenosynovitis. Foot radiographs assist to exclude articular or bony problems. Diagnostic interdigital nerve block of the affected interdigital nerve (usually the third) is confirmatory. Diagnostic ultrasound (US) can be used for diagnosis or to guide therapeutic injection.[13–16] Magnetic resonance imaging (MRI), electrodiagnostic studies (EDX), and bone scan assist primarily in differential diagnosis, and are not universally indicated.[2]

Treatment
Initial treatment includes activity modification, nonsteroidal antiinflammatory drugs (NSAIDs; especially if there is a local synovitis or tenosynovitis), footwear

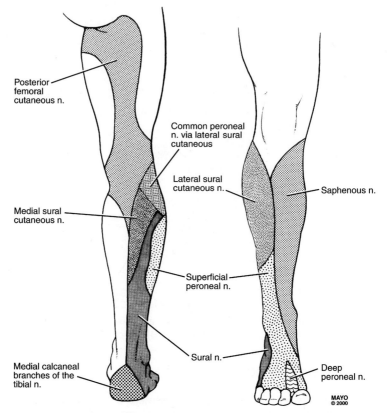

Fig. 7. Cutaneous innervation of the thigh, leg, and foot dorsum. (By permission of Mayo Foundation for Medical Education and Research. All rights reserved.)

modifications, physical therapy, and treating underlying contributing conditions. The athlete may benefit from biomechanical interventions to reduce toe dorsiflexion, control hyperpronation, and maintain greater metatarsal separation. Options include a well-padded supportive sole, a wider shoe, a metatarsal bar or pad (5 to 6 mm), or orthosis. Achilles flexibility should be optimized. Corticosteroids have been used with good results in some case series.[11] Injection complications include MTJ capsular weakening and local adipose and subcutaneous tissue atrophy. Consequently, 1 author suggests avoiding any injections in this region in athletic populations.[10] In refractory cases, some investigators have recommended sonographically guided alcohol ablation of the neuroma, although the efficacy of this intervention has not been specifically studied in athletic populations.[17] Surgery is generally indicated in the presence of a firm clinical diagnosis (usually supported by a diagnostic anesthetic injection) with refractory symptoms. Universally accepted selection criteria do not exist.[2]

TN: Tarsal Tunnel Syndrome

Definition

Tarsal tunnel syndrome (TTS) represents a constellation of processes affecting the TN or its branches at the level of the ankle, producing neuropathic pain along the posteromedial ankle, medial foot, or plantar foot. Among runners, TN entrapment most

Sciatic Nerve	Tibial Nerve	Medial Sural Cutaneous Nerve (MSCN)	
(L4-S3 Spinal	(TN)[a]	Medial Calcaneal Nerve (MCN)[b]	
Segments)		Medial Plantar Nerve (MPN)	Contribution to Third Interdigital Nerve
			Medial Hallucal Nerve
		Lateral Plantar Nerve (LPN)	First Branch of LPN (FB-LPN)[c]
			Contribution to Third Interdigital Nerve
	Common	Lateral Sural Cutaneous Nerve (LSCN)	
	Peroneal Nerve	Superficial Peroneal Nerve (SPN)	
	(CPN)	Deep Peroneal Nerve (DPN)	
Femoral Nerve (FN; L2-4 Spinal Segments)			Saphenous Nerve
Lateral Femoral Cutaneous Nerve (LFCN; L2-3 Spinal Segments)			
Obturator Nerve (ON; L2-4 Spinal Segments)			

[a]Tibial nerve spinal segments at the tarsal tunnel are predominantly S1-S2.

[b]The MCN may arise from the LPN or from the MPN-LPN bifurcation.

[c]May arise directly from the TN; also called the inferior calcaneal nerve, Baxter's nerve, or the nerve to the abductor digiti quinti.

Fig. 8. Neuroanatomy of the lower limb: branching patterns.

commonly occurs at the level of the tarsal tunnel. There is a slight (56%) female predilection.[18] Entrapment of the TN may also occur at the level of the medial gastrocnemius (high TTS), under the fibromuscular arch of the soleus, or as a result of popliteus muscle tear.[2,5,7,9,10,19–21]

Anatomy, pathophysiology, and risk factors

The TN originates from the L4 to S3 spinal segments and is the larger terminal branch of the sciatic nerve.[11] The TN supplies muscular innervation in the posterior thigh and leg, and a cutaneous contribution to the SN, before becoming superficial medial to the Achilles tendon and entering the tarsal tunnel posterior to the medial malleolus (see **Fig. 3**).

The tarsal tunnel is a fibro-osseous space formed by the flexor retinaculum, medial calcaneus, posterior talus, distal tibia, and medial malleolus, and extends from the distal tibia to the navicular bone. Contents include the posterior tibialis (PT) tendon, flexor digitorum longus (FDL) tendon, flexor hallucis longus (FHL) tendon, and tibial neurovascular bundle. The flexor retinaculum spans a distance from 2 cm above to 2 cm below/distal to a line drawn from the center of the medial malleolus to the calcaneal tuberosity, the medial malleolar-calcaneal line.[18]

Over 90% of the time, the TN will divide into the MPN and LPN within the tarsal tunnel, typically at the medial malleolar-calcaneal line.[18] Within 1 to 2 cm below/distal to the medial malleolar-calcaneal line, the MPN and LPN enter separate fibro-osseous canals at the origin of the abductor hallucis muscle (AHM).[5,22] At this point, the LPN may be particularly vulnerable to injury because of its more proximal and oblique course.[18] TTS can involve the TN, MPN, LPN, and at times the medial calcaneal nerve (MCN); consequently, a variety of distinct clinical syndromes may be possible. The common feature is a process arising within the tarsal tunnel.[2]

Five broad etiologic categories for TTS exist: (1) trauma (contusion, ill-fitting foot-wear), (2) compression by space-occupying lesions (eg, venous stasis, ganglion, teno-synovitis, os trigonum, tumors, bone fragments, accessory calf muscles), (3) systemic disease, (4) biomechanical (excessive pronation, joint hypermobility), and (5) idio-pathic.[2,22–30] Repetitive trauma in the setting of predisposing malalignments is most common in runners.[18] Hyperpronation increases AHM tension and may entrap the TN or plantar nerves.[18] Compression from stiff orthoses or space-occupying lesions such as an os trigonum, tenosynovitis, tumor, or ganglion are less common. A specific cause may be identified in 60% to 80% of cases.[18]

Symptoms and signs

The athlete typically describes cramping, burning, and tingling at the medial ankle, medial foot, and/or plantar foot, beyond the limits of tendon and joint anatomic struc-tures. Diffuse foot pain has been reported. Although proximal radiation may be seen in one-third of cases, the medial heel is usually spared because of the proximal origin of the MCN (see next section).[18] Symptoms increase with standing, walking, and running, and decrease with rest, elevation, and loose footwear use. Running on a banked surface promotes hyperpronation and may aggravate symptoms.[11] Rest pain and night pain may occur in provocative positions, and shaking the foot or walking may provide relief, similar to carpal tunnel syndrome.[5,7] Weakness and sensory loss are uncommon, and TTS is rarely bilateral.[2]

Examination includes inspection for malalignment, deformity, and muscular atrophy causing or resulting from TTS, such as forefoot pronation, claw toe, talipes calcaneus, or calcaneovalgus. Palpate all structures along the medial ankle and foot for ganglia, tenosynovitis, and neoplasms. Nerve palpation and percussion testing is completed over the TN and all its terminal branches; a Valleix phenomenon may be elicited.[31] Provocative maneuvers include sustained passive eversion or great toe dorsiflexion to stretch affected nerves, and postexercise examination. With palpation, percussion testing, or provocative maneuvers, symptom reproduction is crucial.

Intrinsic muscular atrophy may be observed, but weakness is difficult to test and uncommon. In severe cases, weakness of toe plantar flexion manifests by reduced push-off on the affected side.[11] Diminished sweat secretion or mild sensory loss may rarely occur on the sole. Ankle instability should be evaluated and could contribute to TTS in runners. A complete spine and lower limb examination is neces-sary to assist in differential diagnosis.[2]

Differential diagnosis and evaluation

Differential diagnosis includes not only alternative diagnoses but also consideration of processes that produce nerve entrapment at the tarsal tunnel. Clinicians should consider polyneuropathy; proximal neuropathy (including double crush injuries from radiculopathy or sciatic neuropathy); distal neuropathy; deep posterior compartment syndrome; popliteal artery entrapment; vascular claudication; venous disease; teno-synovitis or ganglia; plantar fasciitis; tibiotalar or subtalar synovitis, instability or arthritis; and osseous compression.[32,33]

Physical examination helps to differentiate proximal TN injuries. TN injury just distal to the SN contribution spares lateral calcaneal and foot sensation and gastrocnemius-soleus function. Injury distal to the midportion of the leg affects plantar sensation and results in claw toe deformity caused by imbalance between the affected foot intrinsic and the unaffected FDL and extensor digitorum brevis (EDB) muscles.[11] Prominent numbness and tingling, night pain, proximal radiation, and lack of pain during the first few steps in the morning differentiate TTS from plantar fasciitis, although the conditions can coexist.[2,34]

TTS is primarily a clinical diagnosis, although treatment may be dictated by supportive diagnostic studies. Radiographs may reveal osseous compressive lesions or ankle-foot malalignments (weight-bearing views). In the absence of bony anomalies, MRI is effective for examining the tarsal tunnel and reveals an inflammatory lesion or mass in up to 88% of patients with a firm clinical diagnosis of TTS.[35] Diagnostic US can also effectively visualize structures within the tarsal tunnel and accurately identify compressive mass lesions and/or focal changes in TN cross-sectional area.[30,36,37] In acute TTS or in failed nonoperative management, advanced imaging is recommended to determine the presence of synovitis or a space-occupying lesion, and dictate further treatment. Laboratory testing is not universally necessary, but may assist in excluding systemic disease affecting nerves (eg, diabetes, thyroid disease, pernicious anemia) and rheumatologic disorders. EDX studies assist to exclude alternative neurologic disorders. They may be positive in up to 90% of patients with well-established tarsal tunnel syndrome, but do not correlate with surgical findings or clinical outcome.[38] EDX can also be difficult to interpret in TTS, because an increase in spontaneous activity can be seen in normal subjects in the AHM.[2,39]

Treatment

Investigators have recently recommended that a firm diagnosis of TTS be made only when the following triad exists: (1) foot pain and paresthesias, (2) positive nerve percussion sign/Tinel sign, and (3) positive EDX studies. If only 2 exist, the term probable TTS is recommended, and if only 1 exists, the diagnosis should be reconsidered.[18]

Nonoperative treatment is initially warranted in almost all athletes, and is most successful in those with tenosynovitis or contributory flexible foot deformities. Treatment includes activity modification, NSAIDs, neuromodulatory medications (tricyclic and antiepileptic medications), physical therapy, and biomechanical interventions. Physical therapy includes (1) strengthening the foot instrinsic and medial arch supporting muscles, (2) Achilles stretching in subtalar neutral, (3) lower limb kinetic chain rehabilitation, and (4) proprioceptively enriched rehabilitation in cases of ankle or subtalar joint instability.[2,18]

Biomechanical management varies with clinical presentation. Pronation control may be assisted by use of a motion control shoe, medial heel wedge, medial sole wedge/medial buttress, ankle stirrup brace, or fixed ankle walking brace. If symptoms are reproduced by dorsiflexion, temporary use of a heel lift (in combination with appropriate stretching) may be useful. In severe deformities, medial wedges and arch supports may exacerbate symptoms, and more rigid immobilization via a molded hindfoot orthosis, ankle-foot orthosis, or walking boot/cast is usually necessary to maintain the hindfoot in a neutral position. Temporary crutch-assisted weight bearing may be required. In runners with minor, recurrent symptoms, a change in running habits to reduce TN tension may be useful.[2,40]

Treatment should address contributing underlying systemic conditions, local tenosynovitis, venous congestion, or chronic edema. A well-placed corticosteroid injection at the entrapment site may produce excellent results, provided that the PT tendon is avoided and a period of postinjection protected weight bearing is implemented.[18] Injections directed around the TN have been shown to be more accurate with US guidance.[2,41]

Surgery may be indicated when the clinical diagnosis is probable or firm and the athlete has endured several months of debilitating symptoms unresponsive to appropriate nonoperative treatment.[18] Up to 65% of patients (not confined to runners) required surgical treatment in 1 study.[42] Postoperatively, neuropathic symptoms generally improve after 6 weeks, but maximal recovery may take 6 months or more.[7] Although traditionally good or excellent results were reported in 79% to 95% of cases, another more methodologically stringent study indicated only 44% of patients significantly benefited at a minimum 24-month follow-up.[18,43] The investigators concluded that decompression should only be considered when an associated lesion is identified to be in or near the tarsal tunnel by MRI and/or EDX testing; patients with previous ankle-foot surgery, plantar fasciitis, or inflammatory systemic disease should be managed nonoperatively for extended time periods.[18,43]

Endoscopic techniques exist, but concerns have been raised regarding the ability to adequately decompress the affected structures.[22] In cases where ankle or subtalar instability exists, reconstruction should be considered in addition to decompression.[2]

First Branch of the LPN

Definition

Isolated LPN entrapments are relatively rare. Baxter reported 2 cases, both of which occurred after plantar fascia release.[2,9,10] This syndrome seems to be uncommon among runners. More commonly, entrapment specifically affects the FB-LPN, sometimes called the Baxter nerve, the nerve to the abductor digiti quinti muscle, or the inferior calcaneal nerve. FB-LPN entrapment results in neuropathic pain along the medial heel, and less commonly the lateral foot. FB-LPN entrapment is reported to be the most common neurologic cause of heel pain.[9] Up to 15% of athletes with chronic, unresolving heel pain may have FB-LPN entrapment, with runners and joggers accounting for most cases.[5] The average age of runners in the largest series to date was 38 years, and 88% were men.[2,9]

Anatomy, pathophysiology, and risk factors

Within the tarsal tunnel, the FB-LPN usually arises from the LPN, but in 46% of cases it may originate directly from the TN (see **Fig. 3**).[2,22] After penetrating the AHM and its fascia, the FB-LPN courses inferiorly, passing between the deep taut fascia of the AHM medially and the medial caudal margin of the medial head of the quadratus plantae muscle laterally.[9] The nerve then abruptly turns laterally and courses toward the lateral foot between the flexor digitorum brevis and quadratus plantae muscles (see **Fig. 4**).[2]

The FB-LPN ramifies into 3 terminal branches supplying the flexor digitorum brevis, the medial calcaneal periosteum, and abductor digiti quinti. The branch to the calcaneal periosteum often supplies branches to the long plantar ligament as well as an inconsistent branch to the quadratus plantae muscle.[5] There is no cutaneous innervation.

The actual site of FB-LPN entrapment remains controversial, but perhaps most commonly occurs at the site of direction change from an inferior to lateral course deep to the AHM.[9] In this tight space, the FB-LPN may be compressed during pronation when the AHM and quadratus plantae muscle are forced together. Other investigators propose that entrapment may occur in the osteomuscular canal between the calcaneus and the flexor digitorum brevis muscle at the level of the medial anterior corner of the calcaneal tuberosity, or at the plantar aspect of long plantar ligament.[44] FB-LPN entrapment has also been reported secondary to AHM or quadratus plantae hypertrophy, accessory muscles, abnormal bursae, venous varicosities, calcaneal spurs, and scar tissue from adjacent repetitive injury.[2,9,10,44–46]

The FB-LPN lies deep to the plantar fascia origin and the typical site of calcaneal spurs, which typically lie within the flexor digitorum brevis muscle. Because of the FB-LPN's proximity to the plantar fascia, neural irritation is believed to occur in up to 15% to 20% of cases of chronic plantar fasciitis.[2,7,9–11,44] Patients who have proximal edema of the flexor digitorum brevis and edema or microtears in the plantar fascia may be more susceptible.[11] It must be emphasized that this represents only a small portion of the 5% to 10% of individuals with chronic refractory plantar fasciitis. Lying within 5 mm anterior to the calcaneus, the FB-LPN may be injured by a large or fractured calcaneal spur, or iatrogenically during spur removal.[2,6]

Symptoms and signs

The diagnosis of FB-LPN entrapment is primarily clinical. The athlete typically complains of chronic, neuropathic, medial heel pain, often diagnosed as plantar fasciitis. Symptoms are precipitated by sports in 50% of cases.[9] Up to 25% of patients have severe pain in the morning secondary to venous engorgement, but night pain is rare.[6]

According to Baxter and Pfeiffer, the pathognomonic sign of FB-LPN entrapment is maximal pain elicited over the entrapment site on the medial heel, superior to the plantar fascia origin, along a line drawn parallel to the posterior tibia (see **Fig. 3**).[5] In 1 study, 100% of patients exhibited maximal pain over this site, although 42% also had mild tenderness of plantar fascia origin.[9] Positive percussion testing has been reported in only 17% of 53 patients (63 heels) in 1 study.[9] In severe cases, small toe abduction may be limited, or atrophy of the lateral foot muscles may be seen. There are no sensory or reflex deficits.[2]

Differential diagnosis and evaluation

Differential diagnosis is similar to TTS, with the addition of local pathologies. Heel pain syndrome, plantar fasciitis, and fat pad disorders are suggested by finding maximal tenderness in the plantar calcaneal region, anterior medial calcaneus, or mid-medial edge of the plantar fascia, respectively.[2,9] These conditions may coexist with FB-LPN entrapment. Sensory loss on the medial heel suggests a disorder affecting the MCN, L4 radiculopathy, plexopathy, or more diffuse neurologic disease; FB-LPN entrapment does not cause sensory loss.

Diagnostic studies are not uniformly helpful. Radiographic bone spurs are seen in 50% of cases, but are not believed to cause entrapment in most cases. MRI or EDX may be helpful to confirm the diagnosis. In 27 patients with 38 symptomatic heels from surgically documented FB-LPN entrapment, only 44% had involvement of the lateral plantar nerve on EDX testing.[2,6]

Treatment

Most cases of FB-LPN entrapment respond to nonoperative measures following treatment principles used for insertional plantar fasciitis or primary heel pain syndrome.[44] Recommended interventions include activity modification, NSAIDs, and physical therapy and biomechanical management for pronation control. Success has been reported using heel cups with or without a lift, foot strappings, foot orthoses (flexible or rigid), padding, soft-soled shoes, and stretching exercises for the Achilles tendon and plantar fascia.[44] Physical therapy should focus on muscle rebalancing about the ankle-foot and entire lower limb kinetic chain. Neuromodulatory medications (tricyclics and antiseizure medications) and local corticosteroid injections may be useful. One author recommends that no more than 3 injections at 2- to 4-week intervals be attempted.[11] Currently, no prospective trials exist to recommend 1 treatment, or a combination of treatments, over another.[2]

Surgery is indicated for refractory cases and is often based on diagnosis by clinical examination and exclusion of alternative conditions. Most investigators advocate at least 6 to 12 months of nonoperative care before considering surgery. Postoperative recovery typically takes 3 to 6 months, but may be longer if small toe abduction is weak preoperatively.[7] When athletes are carefully selected and the diagnosis is firm, good or excellent results may be seen in approximately 85% of patients.[2,9]

MPN: Jogger's Foot

Definition
Classically, jogger's foot describes a syndrome of neuropathic pain radiating along the medial heel and longitudinal arch resulting from local entrapment of the MPN.[2,40] There is no age or gender predilection.[5]

Anatomy, pathophysiology, and risk factors
After the MPN and LPN exit the tarsal tunnel, each nerve enters a fibro-osseous canal bounded superiorly by the calcaneonavicular or spring ligament and inferiorly by the attachment of the AHM to the navicular bone. The MPN then enters the sole of the foot, passes superficial to the traversing FDL tendon at the Master Knot of Henry, and continues distally along the FHL tendon to divide into terminal medial and lateral branches at the level of the base of the first metatarsal.[5] These branches ramify and terminate as 3 common plantar digital nerves within the medial 3 web spaces. The MPN is a mixed sensorimotor nerve providing sensation to the medial sole and plantar aspect of the first to third and medial fourth toes, as well as motor innervation to the AHM, flexor hallucis brevis, flexor digitorum brevis, and first lumbrical muscles (see **Figs. 3** and **5**).[2]

MPN entrapment typically occurs at the AHM fibro-osseous canal or Master Knot of Henry.[10] The MPN may be compressed externally from orthoses or footwear, or internally by AHM tension.[40] Specific causes include AHM hypertrophy, functional hyperpronation (eg, calcaneovalgus), and high-arched orthoses.[10] A history of previous ankle injuries with instability is common. Jogger's foot has also been reported in association with hallux rigidus, for which it is hypothesized that AHM and flexor digitorum brevis muscle spasm resulted from an unconscious desire to splint the first MTJ from dorsiflexing.[2,5]

Symptoms and signs
The athlete typically reports exercise-induced neuropathic pain radiating along the medial arch toward the plantar aspect of the first and second toes. Symptoms may coincide with implementation of new footwear or an orthosis. There is typically no rest or night pain.

Examination should follow general principles. The most useful palpatory finding is maximal tenderness at the superior aspect of the AHM at the navicular tuberosity, with distally radiating pain or tingling; this site is distinct from that described for FB-LPN entrapment (see **Fig. 3**).[11,40] Provocative testing includes forceful passive heel eversion, standing on the balls of the feet, or percussion over the nerve. Sensory loss, weakness, and atrophy are rarely reported. Because symptoms may only be induced with exercise, examination may be completely normal unless the athlete is examined after running.[10] The athlete should be examined for ankle instabilities, malalignments, hallux rigidus, AHM hypertrophy, and valgus running mechanics.[2]

Differential diagnosis and evaluation
For diagnostic purposes, the syndrome of MPN entrapment or jogger's foot consists of: (1) burning medial heel pain, (2) longitudinal arch aching, and (3) medial sole

paresthesias.[2,40] Differential diagnosis parallels that of TTS, with the exception of additional local pathologic processes. Because of the proximity of the MPN to the FDL and FHL muscles, distinguishing neuropathic pain from tendinitis may be difficult, and the 2 conditions may coexist.[11] Resisted great toe plantar flexion or passive dorsiflexion induces pain with FHL tendinitis, but not typically with nerve entrapment.[11] Hindfoot and midfoot synovitis and arthritis, as well as stress fractures, should be considered.

Evaluation is similar to TTS. Radiographs are commonly obtained, and bone scans are obtained as necessary. MRI has not been as useful for jogger's foot compared with TTS, but may reveal local midfoot arthritis or tendinopathies at the Master Knot of Henry. Diagnostic US may also be useful, but does not reliably provide firm diagnosis. Electrodiagnostic testing aids in the differential diagnosis but sensitivity varies for detecting abnormalities. Diagnostic nerve block at the entrapment site can be useful.[2]

Treatment

Initial nonoperative treatment is indicated and often successful. Treatment principles parallel those for TTS. Rigid orthoses should be modified, replaced, or removed to avoid MPN compression. Functional hyperpronation may be addressed by medial arch strengthening, kinetic chain rehabilitation, modifying running mechanics (less valgus) or terrain, or altering footwear.[40] Therapeutic injections should avoid direct nerve contact. Surgical release has been successful in refractory cases and is generally a distal extension of the surgery performed for TTS.[2]

CPN

Definition

CPN entrapment typically occurs at the fibular head, proximal to the bifurcation into the SPN and DPN, and produces dorsiflexion weakness and possibly neuropathic pain extending over the anterolateral leg and foot dorsum. It is the most prevalent peroneal nerve injury seen in runners.[2,11,47,48]

Anatomy, pathophysiology, and risk factors

The CPN consists of sensory and motor fibers from the L4 to S2 segments and is the smaller terminal branch of the sciatic nerve (see **Figs. 5–7**). The CPN separates from the sciatic nerve just above the knee, where it supplies innervation to the short head of the biceps femoris muscle (the only thigh muscle innervated by the peroneal nerve) and divides into the SPN and DPN, and lateral sural cutaneous nerve (LSCN) at the level of the fibular head (see **Fig. 8**).[2]

The SPN innervates leg lateral compartment muscles, and then emerges from the lateral compartment by penetrating the crural fascia 10.5 to 12.5 cm proximal to the tip of the lateral malleolus. It supplies sensation to the anterolateral leg, then divides into its terminal medial and intermediate cutaneous branches about 6 cm above the lateral malleolus (see **Figs. 6** and **7**). These branches enter the foot dorsum superficial to the inferior extensor retinaculum and supply sensation to the foot dorsum, including the medial aspect of the first toe, and the adjacent sides of the third and fourth, and fourth and fifth toes (see **Fig. 7**). The DPN traverses the leg's anterior compartment, innervating all the muscles including the peroneus tertius, divides into medial and lateral branches 1 to 2 cm proximal to the ankle, and enters the foot deep to the inferior extensor retinaculum. Its medial branch supplies sensation to the first web space, and its lateral branch innervates the EDB as well as local joints. Up to 20% of individuals may have accessory innervation of the EDB from the SPN.[11]

The CPN is vulnerable to compression at the fibular head because of its superficial location and underlying bone. Reported causes of CPN injury include external compression (knee crossing, bed rest, casts, orthoses), aneurysms, tumors (eg, neurofibroma), tibiofibular joint ganglion, tibiofibular dislocation, fibular head hyper-mobility or dislocation, Baker cyst, generalized ligamentous laxity, genu varum, genu recurvatum, compartment syndrome, stress fracture, fabella syndrome, fascial compression by the edge of the peroneus longus muscle, as a sequelae of ankle sprain, direct ice injury, and as a complication after knee surgery.[2,47–55] Repetitive combined plantar flexion and inversion while running downhill or on uneven surfaces may also produce stretch on the CPN at the fibular head.[2]

Symptoms and signs

The DPN is often more severely affected than the SPN. The athlete may report neuro-pathic symptoms affecting the anterior or anterolateral leg, extending into the dorsal foot and toe web spaces. However, the most common complaint is weakness, most often with ankle dorsiflexion given the propensity for DPN involvement.[11] Conse-quently, the athlete may complain of foot drop, steppage gait, foot slap, or recurrent ankle sprains.

Physical examination may be unremarkable at rest, but palpation for masses, fascial defects, nerve sensitivity, pulses, and tibiofibular problems should be performed. Knee lateral and posterolateral rotatory laxity or instability can produce stretch injury to the CPN or its branches at the fibular head. Leach and colleagues reported that postexercise percussion sensitivity or weakness was detected in all 7 patients with CPN injury who had normal baseline examinations.[2,47]

Differential diagnosis and evaluation

Differential diagnosis includes injury to all neurologic structures contributing to the CPN, compartment syndrome, and focal processes about the knee that can lead to CPN injury. A focal CPN injury would not involve the TN sensorimotor functions, or the cutaneous distribution of the saphenous nerve. Sciatic neuropathy, lumbosacral plexopathy, and L5 radiculopathy may also produce foot drop, but typically produce weakness in nonperoneal innervated muscles (eg, PT), nonperoneal territory sensory loss (eg, plantar foot), and nonperoneal reflex loss (eg, ankle reflex). Multiple sclerosis may present as exercise-induced foot drop, with relatively little pain (Uhthoff phenomenon).

Diagnostic US can be useful in detecting intraneural ganglia and other abnormalities of the CPN.[56] Diagnostic studies may also include radiographs and MRI to exclude compressive mass lesions. EDX studies may be extremely helpful for localization, prognostication, and differential diagnosis. However, EDX abnormalities may only occur after exercise.[2,47]

Treatment

CPN entrapments in runners are often self-limited provided the inciting factor is addressed.[47] If considerable axon loss occurs, recovery may be prolonged and incomplete. Treatment includes patient counseling; nerve protection; neuromodula-tory medications, and transcutaneous electrical nerve stimulation (TENS) for neuro-pathic pain; biomechanical interventions to reduce neural tension; dorsiflexion support (ankle brace, ankle-foot orthosis, or high-top shoes); knee stabilization when necessary; change in running style to avoid excessive varus recurvatum knee moments; and observation. If recovery is prolonged and advanced imaging has not been obtained, strong consideration should be given to MRI or US evaluation with the site dictated by the history, examination, and EDX findings.[47] If the clinical diagnosis is firm and significant axonal damage has not occurred, operative decom-pression usually provides satisfactory results. In 1 small study, 6 of 7 young and middle-aged runners returned to normal activities within 6 weeks of surgical treatment.[2,47]

SPN

Definition
SPN entrapment typically occurs as the nerve penetrates the crural fascia above the ankle, resulting in neuropathic pain in the SPN distribution. Among athletes, the mean age is 28 years, and men and women are equally affected.[2,5]

Anatomy, pathophysiology and risk factors
SPN injury at the site of emergence from the lateral compartment may result from sharp fascial edges, chronic ankle sprains (25% of athletes have a history of trauma), muscular herniation, direct contusive trauma, fibular fracture, edema, varicose veins, wearing tight ski boots or roller blades, biomechanical factors (see section on CPN), and space-occupying lesions such as nerve sheath tumors, lipomas, ganglia, ankle fractures, or as a complication of ankle surgery.[2,57,58] The nerve may also be injured iatrogenically during anterior or lateral compartment release. Up to 10% of affected individuals may have chronic lateral compartment syndrome.[59] The medial branch, intermediate branch, or both, may be affected. Because the terminal cutaneous branches enter the foot dorsal to the extensor retinaculum (see **Fig. 6**), they are not entrapped beneath this tissue. However, tight footwear may externally compress the SPN or either of its 2 terminal branches at the level of the ankle or foot, resulting in distal radiating neuropathic pain.[2]

Symptoms and signs
The athlete typically reports a diffuse ache over the sinus tarsi or dorsolateral foot. One-third report numbness or tingling over the same areas.[4] Symptoms may be limited to a vague, achy distal anterolateral leg discomfort, and proximal radiation has been reported.[2,60] Symptoms typically worsen with weight bearing, are relieved by rest, and do not occur at night.

Examination may reveal percussion tenderness, a fascial defect (60% of patients), or muscular herniation at the exit site approximately 10.5 to 12.5 cm above the ankle. Provocative testing before and after exercise is the most useful clinical indicator of SPN entrapment and includes (1) pressure over the exit site during resisted ankle dorsiflexion-eversion, (2) pressure over the same area during passive plantar flexion combined with inversion, and (3) percussion over the SPN course while passive plantar flexion and inversion are maintained. Pain or paresthesias indicate a positive test and the presence of 2 positive tests strongly supports the diagnosis.[59,61] Sensation may be diminished but is not common.[5] Ankle stability, biomechanical alignment, and dorsal footwear pressures should be examined in all athletes.[2]

Differential diagnosis and evaluation
Differential diagnosis resembles that for CPN and should also consider the various causes of SPN injury specifically. Radiographs and EDX may help, but are often unremarkable. Normal nerve conduction studies recorded at rest do not exclude SPN, and postexercise testing has been advocated when necessary.[2,59] Diagnostic US can trace the course of the SPN to assess for abnormalities.[62] MRI can detect most mass lesions, but may not discern contributory fascial defects. Compartment testing is performed as clinically indicated.[2]

Treatment

Treatment parallels that for CPN entrapment, but may also include corticosteroid injection at the site of emergence from the lateral compartment, ankle instability rehabilitation, myofascial release, and lateral heel wedges to decrease nerve stretch. Footwear modification may be necessary to reduce dorsal pressures at the ankle. In refractory confirmed cases, surgery typically consists of isolated release at the fascial exit site, reduction of muscular herniation, fat nodule resection, and fasciotomy if compartment syndrome is documented. Ankle reconstruction is performed as necessary. In isolated releases, athletes begin gradual return to activity at 2 weeks. In Styf's study, up to 75% of patients remain improved at 18 months follow-up; however, only 4 of 17 patients had unlimited activity, whereas 10 of 17 categorized their activity as improved but still limited.[2,59,61]

DPN: Anterior Tarsal Tunnel Syndrome

Definition

DPN entrapment is also called anterior tarsal tunnel syndrome (ATTS), although all investigators do not agree with this latter designation because there is no distinct fibro-osseous tunnel in this region. This syndrome results from DPN in the vicinity of the extensor retinaculum, resulting in neuropathic pain extending into the dorsomedial foot and first web space (see **Figs. 6** and **7**).[2]

Anatomy, pathophysiology, and risk factors

In the anterior leg compartment, the extensor hallucis longus (EHL) muscle courses in a medial oblique direction. The DPN traverses deep to the extensor retinaculum to course between the EHL and extensor digitorum longus (EDL) tendons at the level of the inferior aspect of the superior extensor retinaculum, approximately 3 to 5 cm above the ankle joint. At the level of the oblique superior band of the inferior extensor retinaculum, about 1 cm above the ankle joint, the DPN forms its terminal lateral and medial branches. The lateral branch innervates the EDB muscle. The medial branch courses distally with the dorsalis pedis artery, passing deep to the oblique inferior medial band of the inferior extensor retinaculum, where it may be entrapped by processes affecting the talonavicular joint.[2,5]

DPN entrapment may occur in several locations, including the inferior aspect of the superior extensor retinaculum where the EHL crosses over the DPN, the inferior extensor retinaculum (ATTS; most common site), and distally where the EDB crosses the DPN in the first intermetatarsal space. In the latter 2 cases, an isolated sensory neuropathy of the medial branch occurs. A variety of processes may entrap the DPN, including trauma (contusion, ankle sprain, or instability), shoe contact pressure (boot top neuropathy; wearing a key under the tongue of the shoe), osteophytic compression (tibiotalar, talonavicular, or first metatarsophalangeal), edema, and synovitis or ganglia arising form adjacent joints or tendons.[2,63–66]

Symptoms and signs

Athletes typically report deep, aching, dorsal midfoot pain and neuropathic symptoms extending into the first web space. Symptoms are worse with activity, prolonged standing, and wearing tight-fitting or high-top or lace-up shoes, and are relieved by rest. Night pain can occur from pressure or prolonged plantar flexion positioning.[2,22]

A detailed history often directs attention to ill-fitting footwear as the probable cause in many cases.[22] Percussion along the course of the DPN starting at the fibular head may localize the entrapment site. Depending on the entrapment site, symptom provocation may occur with either plantar flexion or dorsiflexion of the foot.[10,22] EDB weakness is difficult to detect. Atrophy relative to the unaffected side may be seen, but should not be expected if only the medial branch is involved. Examination should also focus on revealing potential etiologic processes, as discussed later. Biomechanical factors are not as crucial in this nerve entrapment relative to those discussed previously.[2]

Differential diagnosis and evaluation

Differential diagnosis parallels that for CPN and SPN entrapments but also includes anterior compartment syndrome as well as an evaluation for treatable causes of DPN injury. Recall that CPN entrapments often preferentially affect the DPN fascicles, so CPN injury presenting as DPN injury should be excluded.[2,11] Involvement of the EDB localizes injury above the extensor retinaculum.

Radiographs may reveal dorsal midfoot osteophytes or accessory ossicles (eg, os intermetatarseum) that may irritate terminal branches of the DPN.[23] EDX can assist in differential diagnosis and localization (eg, involvement of the EDB or CPN). Compartment pressures, diagnostic US, and MRI are obtained as necessary.[2]

Treatment

Nonoperative measures include footwear changes to avoid direct pressure, neuromodulatory and antiinflammatory medications, TENS, edema control, ankle stability rehabilitation, and local corticosteroid injections. Local injections assist diagnostically and therapeutically. Treatable underlying causes are addressed. Surgery is sometimes necessary, is performed via a dorsomedial approach, and involves partial sectioning of the extensor retinaculum and osteophyte removal. Recovery may take 6 to 8 weeks.[2]

SN

The SN is an uncommon area of neuropathy. There is no particular sex or age distribution, but the syndrome is reported most commonly in runners. The SN is formed by branches of the TN and CPN in the posterior calf, 11 to 20 cm proximal to the lateral malleolus. Two centimeters proximal to the lateral malleolus, the SN provides a sensory branch to the lateral heel, then courses subcutaneously inferior to the peroneal tendons to the base of the fifth metatarsal, where it ramifies into distal sensory branches (see **Figs. 5** and **7**).

Causes include recurrent ankle sprains, calcaneal or fifth metatarsal fractures, Achilles tendinopathy, space-occupying lesions such as ganglia (peroneal sheath, calcaneocuboid joint), direct contusion, footwear-induced pressure, or iatrogenic (postbiopsy neuroma or injury during ankle arthroscopy).[2,67,68] Symptoms consist of achy, posterolateral calf pain, with neuropathic pain in the SN distribution (see **Figs. 5** and **7**). Examination should include percussion testing along the nerve and provocative testing by passive dorsiflexion and inversion. Diagnostic testing is not universally required, but may include radiographs, diagnostic US, EDX, and diagnostic nerve blocks. Treatment emphasizes reduction of pressure from footwear, Achilles stretching, neuropathic pain treatment, edema control, and ankle stability rehabilitation. When SN block is indicated, US guidance has been shown to improve clinical outcome.[69] Etiologic conditions should be identified and treated. Surgery consists of exploration and decompression.[2]

Saphenous Nerve

The saphenous nerve is the largest cutaneous branch of the femoral nerve. This purely sensory nerve arises from the femoral nerve in the femoral triangle and courses with the femoral artery to the medial knee, where its infrapatellar branch supplies cutaneous sensation to the medial knee. It then courses inferiorly with the saphenous vein to supply cutaneous sensation to the medial calf to the level of the ankle.[2,7] At the ankle, a branch passes anterior to the medial malleolus to innervate the medial foot (see **Figs. 3** and **5**). The saphenous nerve is most vulnerable at the medial knee, where it pierces the fascia and emerges from the distal subsartorial canal (Hunter adductor canal). Causes of saphenous neuritis include entrapment at the adductor canal, pes anserine bursitis, contusion, patellar dislocation, postsurgical (knee or ankle) iatrogenic injury, or as a complication related to knee injection.[2,70–75]

The athlete typically reports neuropathic pain and numbness in the area of the medial knee and/or calf, depending on whether there is isolated infrapatellar branch or complete saphenous nerve involvement. Saphenous neuritis related to pes anserine bursitis may clinically resemble tibial stress fracture.[70] There should be no motor deficits. Examination includes percussion testing along the nerve starting at the adductor canal, and a search for underlying causes. Differential diagnosis includes all proximal femoral nerve, plexus, and root lesions, as well as musculoskeletal disorders about the knee. Diagnosis and treatment principles resemble those for SN entrapment, but focus on different anatomic areas. Surgical release or excision of a neuroma[74] may be necessary.

MISCELLANEOUS NERVE ENTRAPMENT SYNDROMES

Although significantly less common among runners, several additional nerve entrapment syndromes may be encountered by clinicians caring for runners, including entrapment of the medial calcaneal, lateral femoral cutaneous, and obturator nerves. Discussions of these entrapment neuropathies are beyond the scope of this article.

REFERENCES

1. Massey E, Pleet A. Neuropathy in joggers. Am J Sports Med 1978;6:209–11.
2. Smith J, Dahm D. Nerve entrapments. In: O'Connor F, Wilder R, editors. The textbook of running medicine. New York: McGraw-Hill; 2001. p. 257–72.
3. Coughlin MJ, Mann RA, Saltzman CL. Surgery of the foot and ankle. 8th edition. St. Louis (MO): Mosby; 2006.
4. Styf J. Chronic exercise induced pain in the anterior aspect of the lower leg: an overview of diagnosis. Sports Med 1989;7:331–9.
5. Schon L, Baxter D. Neuropathies of the foot and ankle in athletes. Clin Sports Med 1990;9:489–509.
6. Schon L, Glennon T, Baxter D. Heel pain syndrome: electrodiagnostic support for nerve entrapment. Foot Ankle 1993;14:129.
7. Schon L. Nerve entrapment, neuropathy, and nerve dysfunction in the athlete. Orthop Clin North Am 1994;25:47–59.
8. Babcock J. Cervical spine injuries: diagnosis and classification. Arch Surg 1976; 111:647–61.
9. Baxter D, Pfeffer G. Treatment of chronic heel pain by surgical release of the first branch of the lateral plantar nerve. Clin Orthop Relat Res 1992;279:299.
10. Baxter D. Functional nerve disorders in the athlete's foot, ankle and leg. Instr Course Lect 1993;42:185–94.
11. McCluskey L, Webb L. Compression and entrapment neuropathies of the lower extremity. Clin Podiatr Med Surg 1999;16:96–125.
12. Wu KK. Morton's interdigital neuroma: a clinical review of its etiology, treatment, and results. J Foot Ankle Surg 1996;35(2):112–9.
13. Sofka C, Adler R. Ultrasound guided interventions in the foot and ankle. Semin Musculoskelet Radiol 2002;6:163–8.

14. Quinn T, Jacobson J, Craig J, et al. Sonography of Morton's neuroma. Am J Roentgenol 2000;174:1723–8.
15. Gregg J, Marks P. Metatarsalgia: an ultrasound perspective. Australas Radiol 2007;51:493–9.
16. Hughes R, Ali K, Jones H, et al. Treatment of Morton's neuroma with alcohol injection under sonographic guidance. Am J Roentgenol 2007;188:1535–9.
17. Hughes RJ, Ali K, Jones H, et al. Treatment of Morton's neuroma with alcohol injection under sonographic guidance: follow-up of 101 cases. Am J Roentgenol 2007;188(6):1535–9.
18. Lau J, Daniels T. Tarsal tunnel syndrome: a review of the literature. Foot Ankle Int 1999;20:201–9.
19. Peri G. The "critical zones" of entrapment of the nerves of the lower limb. Surg Radiol Anat 1991;13(2):139–43.
20. Feinberg JH, Spielholz NI, editors. Peripheral nerve injuries in the athlete. Champaign (IL): Human Kinetics; 2003. p. 106–41.
21. de Ruiter GC, Torchia ME, Amrami KK, et al. Neurovascular compression following isolated popliteus muscle rupture: a case report. J Surg Orthop Adv 2005;14(3):129–32.
22. Park T, DelToro D. Electrodiagnostic evaluation of the foot. Phys Med Rehabil Clin N Am 1998;9:871–96.
23. Murphy P, Baxter D. Nerve entrapment of the foot and ankle in runners. Clin Sports Med 1985;4:753–63.
24. Pla ME, Dillingham TR, Spellman NT, et al. Painful legs and moving toes associated with tarsal tunnel syndrome and accessory soleus muscle. Mov Disord 1996;11(1):82–6.
25. Sammarco GJ, Stephens MM. Tarsal tunnel syndrome caused by the flexor digitorum accessorius longus. A case report. J Bone Joint Surg Am 1990;72(3):453–4.
26. Jackson DL, Haglund B. Tarsal tunnel syndrome in athletes. Case reports and literature review. Am J Sports Med 1991;19(1):61–5.
27. Park TA, Del Toro DR. The medial calcaneal nerve: anatomy and nerve conduction technique. Muscle Nerve 1995;18(1):32–8.
28. Stefko RM, Lauerman WC, Heckman JD. Tarsal tunnel syndrome caused by an unrecognized fracture of the posterior process of the talus (Cedell fracture). A case report. J Bone Joint Surg Am 1994;76(1):116–8.
29. Yamamoto S, Tominaga Y, Yura S, et al. Tarsal tunnel syndrome with double causes (ganglion, tarsal coalition) evoked by ski boots. Case report. J Sports Med Phys Fitness 1995;35(2):143–5.
30. Nagaoka M, Matsuzaki H. Ultrasonography in tarsal tunnel syndrome. J Ultrasound Med 2005;24:1035–40.
31. Dumitru D, Amato AA, Zwarts MJ, editors. Electrodiagnostic medicine. 2nd edition. Philadelphia: Hanley & Belfus; 2001. p. 1103.
32. Sammarco G, Chalk D, Feibel J. Tarsal tunnel syndrome and additional nerve lesions in the same limb. Foot Ankle 1993;14:71–7.
33. Turnipseed W, Pozniak M. Popliteal entrapment as a result of neurovascular compression by the soleus and plantaris muscles. J Vasc Surg 1992;15:285–92.
34. Jackson D, Haglund B. Tarsal tunnel syndrome in runners. Sports Med 1992;13:146–9.
35. Frey C, Kerr R. Magnetic resonance imaging and the evaluation of tarsal tunnel syndrome. Foot Ankle 1993;14:153–64.

36. Vijayan J, Therimadasamy AK, Teoh HL, et al. Sonography as an aid to neurophysiological studies in diagnosing tarsal tunnel syndrome. Am J Phys Med Rehabil 2009;88(6):500–1.

37. Alshami AM, Cairns CW, Wylie BK, et al. Reliability an size of the measurement error when determining cross-sectional area of the tibial nerve at the tarsal tunnel with ultrasonography. Ultrasound Med Biol 2009;35(7):1098–102.

38. Galardi G, Amadio S, Maderna L, et al. Electrophysiologic studies in tarsal tunnel syndrome: diagnostic reliability of motor distal latency, mixed nerve and sensory nerve conduction studies. Am J Phys Med 1994;73:193–8.

39. Boon AJ, Harper CM. Needle EMG of abductor hallucis and peroneus tertius in normal subjects. Muscle Nerve 2003;27(6):752–6.

40. Rask M. Medial plantar neuropraxia (Jogger's foot). Clin Orthop 1978;181: 167–70.

41. Redborg KE, Antonakakis JG, Beach ML, et al. Ultrasound improves the success rate of a tibial nerve block at the ankle. Reg Anesth Pain Med 2009;34(3):256–60.

42. Cimino W. Tarsal tunnel syndrome: review of the literature. Foot Ankle 1990;11: 47–52.

43. Pfeiffer W, Cracchiolo A. Clinical results after tarsal tunnel decompression. J Bone Joint Surg Br 1994;76A:1222–30.

44. Johnson M. Nerve entrapment causing heel pain. Clin Podiatr Med Surg 1994;11: 617–24.

45. Park TA, Del Toro DR. Isolated inferior calcaneal neuropathy. Muscle Nerve 1996; 19(1):106–8.

46. Fredericson M, Standage S, Chou L, et al. Lateral plantar nerve entrapment in a competitive gymnast. Clin J Sport Med 2001;11(2):111–4.

47. Leach R, Purnell M, Saito A. Peroneal nerve entrapment in runners. Am J Sports Med 1989;17:287–91.

48. Moller B, Kadin S. Entrapment of the common peroneal nerve. Am J Sports Med 1987;15:90–1.

49. Di Risio D, Lazaro R, Popp A. Nerve entrapment and calf atrophy caused by a Baker's cyst: case report. Neurosurgery 1994;35:333–4.

50. Nagel A, Greenebaum E, Singson R, et al. Foot drop in a long-distance runner. An unusual presentation of neurofibromatosis. Orthop Rev 1994;23:526–30.

51. Al-Kashmiri A, Delaney JS. Fatigue fracture of the proximal fibula with secondary common peroneal nerve injury. Clin Orthop Relat Res 2007;463:225–8.

52. Dawson DM, Hallett M, Wilbourn AJ, editors. Entrapment neuropathies. 3rd edition. Philadelphia: Lippincott-Raven; 1999. p. 273–8.

53. Meals RA. Peroneal-nerve palsy complicating ankle sprain. Report of two cases and review of the literature. J Bone Joint Surg Am 1977;59(7):966–8.

54. Moeller JL, Monroe J, McKeag DB. Cryotherapy-induced common peroneal nerve palsy. Clin J Sport Med 1997;7(3):212–6.

55. Peicha G, Pascher A, Schwarzl F, et al. Transection of the peroneal nerve complicating knee arthroscopy: case report and cadaver study. Arthroscopy 1998; 14(2):221–3.

56. Visser L. High resolution sonography of the common peroneal nerve: detection of intraneural ganglia. Neurology 2006;67:1473–5.

57. Redfern DJ, Sauve PS, Sakellariou A. Investigation of incidence of superficial peroneal nerve injury following ankle fracture. Foot Ankle Int 2003;24(10): 771–4.

58. Takao M, Ochi M, Shu N, et al. A case of superficial peroneal nerve injury during ankle arthroscopy. Arthroscopy 2001;17(4):403–4.

59. Styf J, Morberg P. The superficial peroneal tunnel syndrome: results of treatment by decompression. J Bone Joint Surg Br 1997;79:801–3.
60. Lowdon I. Superficial peroneal nerve entrapment. J Bone Joint Surg Br 1985;67: 58–9.
61. Styf J. Entrapment of the superficial peroneal nerve: diagnosis and results of decompression. J Bone Joint Surg Br 1989;71:131–5.
62. Canella C, Demondion X, Guillin R, et al. Anatomic study of the superficial peroneal nerve using sonography. Am J Roentgenol 2009;193(1):174–9.
63. Dellon A. Deep peroneal nerve entrapment on the dorsum of the foot. Foot Ankle 1990;11:73–80.
64. Dallari D, Pellacani A, Marinelli A, et al. Deep peroneal nerve paresis in a runner caused by ganglion at capitulum peronei. Case report and review of the literature. J Sports Med Phys Fitness 2004;44(4):436–40.
65. Lindenbaum BL. Ski boot compression syndrome. Clin Orthop Relat Res 1979; 140:109–10.
66. Gessini L, Jandolo B, Pietrangeli A. The anterior tarsal syndrome. Report of four cases. J Bone Joint Surg Am 1984;66(5):786–7.
67. Gould N, Trevino S. Sural nerve entrapment by avulsion fracture of the base of the fifth metatarsal bone. Foot Ankle 1981;2(3):153–5.
68. Nakano KK. Entrapment neuropathy from Baker's cyst. JAMA 1978;239(2):135.
69. Redborg KE, Sites BD, Chinn CD, et al. Ultrasound improves the success rate of a sural nerve block at the ankle. Reg Anesth Pain Med 2009;34(1):24–8.
70. Hemler DE, Ward WK, Karstetter KW, et al. Saphenous nerve entrapment caused by pes anserine bursitis mimicking stress fracture of the tibia. Arch Phys Med Rehabil 1991;72(5):336–7.
71. Gleeson AP, Kerr JG. Patella dislocation neurapraxia - a report of two cases. Injury 1996;27(7):519–20.
72. Ferkl RD, Heath DD, Guhl JF. Neurological complications of ankle arthroscopy. Arthroscopy 1996;12(2):200–8.
73. Logue EJ 3rd, Drez D Jr. Dermatitis complicating saphenous nerve injury after arthroscopic debridement of a medial meniscal cyst. Arthroscopy 1996;12(2): 228–31.
74. Worth RM, Kettelkamp DB, Defalque RJ, et al. Saphenous nerve entrapment. A cause of medial knee pain. Am J Sports Med 1984;12(1):80–1.
75. Iizuka M, Yao R, Wainapel S. Saphenous nerve injury following medial knee joint injection: a case report. Arch Phys Med Rehabil 2005;86(10):2062–5.

Exertional Collapse in the Runner: Evaluation and Management in Fieldside and Office-Based Settings

Marc A. Childress, MD[a],*, Francis G. O'Connor, MD, MPH[b], Benjamin D. Levine, MD[c]

KEYWORDS

- Sudden death • Exercise-related syncope
- Exertional collapse • Normothermia

As the popularity of recreational and competitive running continues to increase, greater attention is being paid to certain aspects of medical care for runners, both individually and in the context of mass participation events. One area of particular interest has been of exertional collapse in a runner, defined as the inability to stand or walk unaided as a result of lightheadedness, faintness, dizziness, or syncope. Runners, spectators, and medical personnel identify with the common occurrence of this phenomenon, particularly in the context of higher intensity and longer distance events.[1] In addition, recent lay literature has recorded numerous collapses resulting in sudden death events, with many occurring in young adults.[2,3] This discussion explores the epidemiology, pathophysiology, and the broad differential diagnosis of collapse in a runner, as well as evaluation and treatment strategies for acute fieldside and nonacute office-based assessments.

DEFINITIONS

Because exertional collapse does not represent a singular medical diagnosis, it is helpful to define some of the associated conditions that are pertinent in the following

[a] Department of Family and Sports Medicine, DeWitt Army Community Hospital, Fort Belvoir, VA, USA
[b] Department of Military and Emergency Medicine, Consortium for Health and Military Performance, Uniformed Services University of the Health Sciences, Bethesda, MD, USA
[c] Institute for Exercise and Environmental Medicine, Presbyterian Hospital, University of Texas Southwestern Medical Center, Dallas, TX, USA
* Corresponding author.
E-mail address: Marc.childress@amedd.army.mil

Clin Sports Med 29 (2010) 459–476
doi:10.1016/j.csm.2010.03.007
0278-5919/10/$ – see front matter. Published by Elsevier Inc.

discussion. Exercise-associated collapse (EAC) is a term used to describe an athlete with an inability to stand or walk secondary to lightheadedness, faintness, dizziness, or syncope. EAC is not a clinical diagnosis but rather a chief complaint. In some cases, a medical diagnosis such as heat stroke or cardiac arrest secondary to an acute myocardial infarction may be identified. The literature, however, has adopted the term, EAC, to represent and define those cases of collapse whereby no other specific cause is identified. In practical terms, EAC is more often used to distinguish an episode of collapse after stopping prolonged or intense activity because of the sudden decrease in venous return on relaxation of the skeletal muscles. While not always true, EAC victims may be able to assist in their own care. EAC excludes orthopedic injuries, for example, sprained ankle or leg cramps, which would preclude completing an event.[4]

Syncope is defined as a transient loss of consciousness secondary to cerebral hypoperfusion followed by spontaneous recovery. Presyncope has a similar mechanism of cerebral hypoperfusion, but the symptoms would include lightheadedness or dizziness that did not fully manifest in a loss of consciousness. Although these conditions are common and widely discussed in the medical literature, their occurrence during exercise may be a harbinger of more significant underlying disease. Runners and other athletes are no less susceptible to the same underlying causes of syncope or presyncope seen at rest or in any sedentary population. However, numerous studies have correlated exertional syncope with a higher risk for cardiovascular disease.[5,6] Conditions such as hypertrophic cardiomyopathy, coronary artery anomalies, long QT syndrome (LQTS), and arrhythmogenic right ventricular cardiomyopathy may first manifest as syncope/presyncope and subsequent collapse during exercise.[7–9] To highlight these distinct concerns associated with syncope or presyncope occurring in the context of exercise, the term exercise-related syncope (ERS) is used to specify these episodes that might occur during or immediately after activity.

These terms do not describe exclusive phenomenon, and caution should be taken in making treatment and evaluation decisions rapidly based on assumptions about any of these conditions. In the acute management of exertional collapse, the need for a specific diagnosis is less important than the need for rapidly assessing the possibility of high-morbidity conditions. In the postevent clinical setting, it is often difficult to easily test for and diagnose every potential condition. Thus, much of the effort in a clinical setting is directed at the potential of underlying cardiac pathology. The following discussion and accompanying algorithms offer a suggested manner in which patients can be evaluated, both in the acute setting such as a mass participation event and in the postevent clinical setting.

EPIDEMIOLOGY

Although it is difficult to establish solid epidemiologic data on collapse in a broad and varied population such as runners, the information collected from mass participation events has proved to be helpful in focusing on the largest areas of concern. Much of this data is from longer endurance events such as marathons and triathlons, with certain themes appearing to be consistent with these reviews (**Box 1**). Although the epidemiologic literature identifies EAC as multifactorial, certain risk factors such as race duration, temperature, gender, and race completion time offer important clinical clues to the sports medicine provider.

In addition to the risk factors described earlier, it is clear that the location of the EAC event on the course in relation to the finish line is an important discriminator for the cause of exertional collapse. Holtzausen and colleagues[10] first commented on this

---

Box 1
EAC: conclusions from the literature

- Medical tent visits increase as the distance of the race increases
- The majority of medical complaints, including collapse, occur at the finish line
- Collapse during the race is often more ominous than collapse occurring at the finish line
- Risks for certain conditions increase along predictable patterns
  - Hyponatremia rates increase with longer race distance
  - Heat illness (HI) rate increases with higher race start temperatures
  - The overall risk of sudden death during running events is small

---

observation when describing the characteristics of collapsed ultramarathoners. These investigators confirmed anecdotal observations that while the majority of athletes collapse at the finish line or in the finish line chute, collapse on the course generally identifies a more serious illness. The biochemical analysis of collapsed athletes versus control athletes did not demonstrate significant differences when looking at the state of hydration, suggesting that the mechanism of collapse is multifactorial and not simply the result of dehydration.

Race duration is varied directly with the number of potential medical encounters. Hiller[11] was the first to note this association in the triathlon community. He reported on medical encounters in 6 triathlons including the Hawaii Ironman. The first observation is that as the race distance increases, so do the tent visits; there is a 2% casualty rate at Olympic distance, with up to 17% at Ironman events. With longer events, hyponatremia also seemed to be a more prevalent problem. At both events, dehydration and heat exhaustion were the most frequent diagnoses. In a subsequent review of Ironman data from 1981 to 1988 Laird,[12] long-time Medical Director of the Hawaii Ironman, confirmed the trends in the Hiller article that longer events generate more casualties. He also noted that 71% of the casualties at the event occur at the finish line. In a 12-year review of marathon data, Roberts,[13] Medical Race Director of the Twin Cities Marathon, studied 81,277 entrants from 1982 to 1994. The finish area medical encounter rates for marathon runners were 18.9 per 1000 entrants and 25.3 per 1000 finishers. Mild injury/illness accounted for 90% of finish line medical encounters: EAC (59%), skin problems (21%), musculoskeletal problems (17%), and other medical problems (3%). Of this group, only 112 runners received intravenous fluids, with 30 runners requiring transfer to emergency medical facilities.

Epidemiologic data have confirmed that perhaps the most important determinant of collapse during a race event is environmental temperature. Roberts reviewed data from the Boston and Twin Cities Marathons and found that finish line encounters and course dropouts increase as conditions deviate from the most advantageous conditions in the 4.4°C to 15°C (40°F–59°F) wet bulb globe temperature (WBGT) range. The risk of requiring medical attention and not finishing increases considerably when the WBGT is more than 15.5°C (60°F). In addition, correlation coefficients of the data suggest that the risks of medical problems and not finishing are associated with the warmest temperature of the race and not the start temperature.[14]

It has been the senior author's (F.G.O'C.) experience that race duration is additionally a predictive element in EAC epidemiology. In a 2004 Marine Corps Marathon competitors study, the investigators analyzed 40 finish line cases of EAC.[15] The race started at 8:15 AM with 22,666 runners, with a low temperature of 60.8°F and a high temperature of 78.8°F. There were 16,400 finishers with 40 patients treated in the finish line tent for collapse; 38 of these 40 subjects finished the race. The average finish time was 4 hours 30 minutes and the average age was 38 years; 25 were men and 15 were women. Diagnoses included 25 with EAC, 4 with exercise-associated muscle cramps, 5 with exertional hyponatremia, and 6 with exertional HI. Hyponatremia was more common in women ($P = .035$), whereas intravenous therapy was used more in patients with HI ($P<.001$) and hyponatremia ($P = .0112$) than in EAC. Transfers were more common with HI ($P<.001$) and hyponatremia ($P<.001$) than in EAC. HI was more common in earlier finishers (3:29 ± 0:24), whereas hyponatremia tended to occur more commonly in later finishers (4:49 ± 0:49).

Although sudden death events are uncommon, they are the most feared cause of EAC among runners and medical providers. Maron and colleagues[16] first reported on the incidence of sudden death at the Marine Corps Marathon and the Twin Cities Marathon. In this review, 215,413 runners completed the marathons with 4 exercise-related sudden deaths occurring; 3 during the race, 1 right after event completion. The investigators concluded that the death rate is small (1 in 50,000), which is in fact one-hundredth the risk of general living for a 1-year period, and probably does not justify the need for medical releases. In a subsequent update, Roberts and Maron[17] reestimated the death rate as 1 in 220,000 marathon race entrants.

With these factors as background, there exists a fairly consistent group of diagnoses associated with collapse during running and/or prolonged exercise (**Box 2**), including focal orthopedic and musculoskeletal complaints, metabolic abnormalities, and cardiopulmonary conditions. For medical personnel who may care for collapsed runners during or after the event, it is helpful to maintain this broad differential and pursue appropriate diagnosis and treatment in an efficient and systematic manner.

PATHOPHYSIOLOGY

To better understand the trends described earlier in the context of collapse, it is necessary to have a basic knowledge of the pertinent physiology. Even at the simplest level, the ability to maintain upright motion requires a complex interplay of muscular regulation, skeletal and soft tissue support, and the maintenance of adequate amounts of oxygen and fuel supplies. It is generally self-evident how

---

Box 2
Conditions associated with collapse during or after prolonged exercise

EAC

   Cardiac arrest

Muscle cramps

   Asthma exacerbation

Heat stroke

   Anaphylaxis

Hyponatremia

   Orthopedic conditions

Hypoglycemia

   Other medical conditions

Hypothermia

conditions such as hypoglycemia, systemic hypoxia (ie, asthma exacerbation), and focal musculoskeletal complaints can inhibit one's ability to stay upright and in motion. There also tends to be a relative understanding of the cardiac physiology and how the "supply and demand" principle can be used to explain the manifestation of cardiac ischemia, structural abnormalities, and arrhythmias. The role and effect of cardiovascular regulation during exercise and how these changes can be the causative factor in many episodes of exertional collapse become less obvious.[18] **Fig. 1** demonstrates a physiologic approach to the differential for ERS/presyncope that highlights these factors.

During aerobic exercise, blood is selectively shunted away from nonexercising areas and directed to active muscles, resulting in a displacement away from the heart and central vasculature. When this happens, the requirement of the heart to have adequate venous return is maintained in great part by the contraction and increased venous pressure of the skeletal muscles. The skeletal muscle becomes, in effect, a second heart. As the muscular pressure changes, venous return can be maintained by relative vasoconstriction. For athletes, numerous adaptations may further complicate this pattern. In well-trained patients, there may be an increased resting parasympathetic tone that can attenuate an expected sympathetic response to a perceived hypovolemia, blunting the vasoconstriction response.[19] It has also been shown that athletes have a higher incidence of syncope during lower body negative pressure testing, possibly reflecting a larger volume capacity in the lower extremities of athletes.[20]

FIELDSIDE MANAGEMENT

In the acute setting, the ability to immediately determine the urgency and general scope of the situation is of paramount importance. This judgment can be further

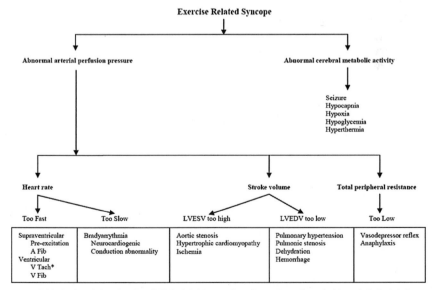

*Etiologies of ventricular tachycardia or fibrillation include hypertrophic cardiomyopathy, arrythmogenic right ventricular dysplasia, long QT syndrome, drugs, structural defects, ion channel disorders, cardiomyopathy, ischemia, etc.

LVESV: left ventricular end systolic volume; LVEDV: left ventricular end diastolic volume; A Fib: atrial fibrillation; V Tach: ventricular tachycardia; V Fib: ventricular fibrillation.

Fig. 1. Differential diagnosis of ERS in athletes.

complicated by the potential of mass participation events to result in a large number of casualties in a short amount of time; comparisons are frequently made to a mass casualty scenario. The ability of on-scene providers to appropriately triage, assess, and provide appropriate initial treatment is critical. The fieldside portion of this discussion focuses on a series of algorithms that have been developed for use in managing emergencies during mass participation events. Specifically, they have been used in conjunction with the Marine Corps Marathon and reflect an attempt to efficiently and appropriately manage collapsed athletes.[21,22] These algorithms demonstrate a practical pattern for the evaluation of the collapsed athlete, in the context of the most likely conditions and the most worrisome conditions.

As **Fig. 2** suggests, the initial assessment is the patient's responsiveness. An unresponsive athlete should be treated in a manner consistent with current advanced cardiovascular life support recommendations, including rapid evaluation of the airway, breathing, and circulation, as well as appropriate use of an automatic external defibrillator. In any situation involving an unresponsive athlete, EMS should be activated immediately. Even the best-equipped medical tent is a less than ideal location to pursue prolonged cardiopulmonary resuscitation. Individual providers and organizers of group support for mass participation events should develop specific plans to deal with cardiac emergencies in accordance with these guidelines and available resources.

The remainder of the collapsed athlete algorithm (see **Fig. 2**) outlines a stepwise assessment that can help readily identify patients who may need aggressive assistance. For responsive patients, a brief history is critical. The brief history includes recall from the patient as well as any available bystander accounts. A focused and pertinent physical examination should be performed, including an accurate set of vital signs. It is helpful to remember that during this initial history taking and examination, it is imperative that the patient's mental status be assessed. Any alteration in mentation or level of consciousness can be a critical factor in deciding the curative care for several conditions that may be encountered in a collapsed athlete. After this point of rapid evaluation, any clearly identifiable medical emergency such as overt signs of anaphylaxis, asthma exacerbation, or focal orthopedic or musculoskeletal complaints should be identified and treated accordingly. For patients without clear signs of an easily identifiable condition that would explain an episode of collapse, it is first recommended that a rectal temperature be obtained. A patient with an identified rectal temperature of greater than 40°C should be diverted immediately for rapid cooling, during or after which other necessary evaluations may be pursued. Patients who are essentially normothermic, within the range of 36°C to 40°C, can be further evaluated according to the EAC algorithm (**Fig. 3**). For patients who demonstrate a rectal temperature of less than 36°C, care can be administered according to the recommendations described below regarding hypothermia.

Taken as a whole, **Fig. 2** (The Collapsed Athlete Algorithm) illustrates a practical fashion by which acutely collapsed patients can be quickly and appropriately classified based on an immediate assessment of responsiveness, available event history, and reliable vital signs. The resultant branches of this parent algorithm allow for more definitive evaluation, and care recommendations are discussed in this article briefly on an individual basis. More exhaustive recommendations are available online at http://champ.usuhs.mil/chclinicaltools.html.

Once a patient has been found to be responsive and without signs of readily identifiable medical problems as described earlier, it is recommended that a rectal temperature be obtained. Although there are many options for obtaining body temperature that may be more palatable to the patient and provider, it is important to point out

Management of the Collapsed Endurance Athlete

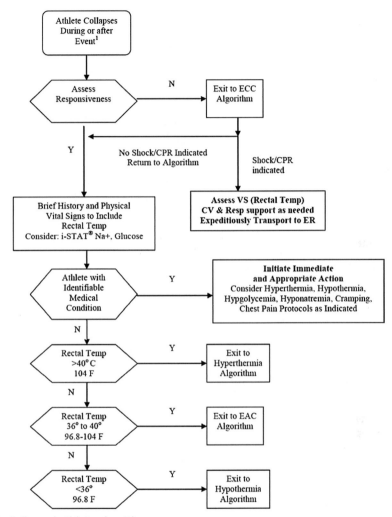

Fig. 2. Collapsed athlete algorithm.

that other means are markedly inconsistent in measuring core temperature.[23,24] This variability may be further exaggerated in the context of exertion and exercise. The presence of altered mental status in athletes found to have a core temperature greater than or equal to 40°C (104°F) meets the conventional definition of exertional heat stroke.[25] In these instances, rapid cooling is the paramount concern. Although the literature describes many options for achieving rapid cooling, ice-water immersion has shown to be consistently the most efficient at achieving a lowered temperature.[26] While cooling, intravenous fluids can be administered, and basic studies for hyponatremia and hypoglycemia can be obtained if available. Ice-water cooling should be continued until the temperature reaches 38.5°C to 39°C, and the patient should be removed from immersion to prevent iatrogenic hypothermia. Patients who are not

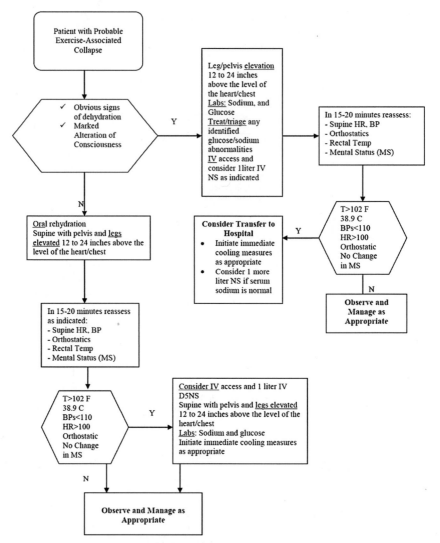

Fig. 3. EAC algorithm. BP, blood pressure; HR, heart rate; IV, intravenous; NS, normal saline.

responding to cooling within 15 to 20 minutes should be prepared for transport, while all possible cooling measures are continued. If ice-water immersion is not feasible, alternative means for cooling can include temperate water immersion; packaged ice in the axilla, neck, and groin; misting fans; cool water application; and covering the patient with wet sheets.[26,27] Even in patients who show an appropriate response to cooling, including a normalization of mentation, they should be transported to a medical facility for further evaluation to assess for evidence of rhabdomyolysis or end-organ damage.

Although it is most likely that the conditions of the day would increase the likelihood of one extreme of environmental exposures, namely heat illness versus cold injury, it is not impossible that both conditions could be encountered in the same setting. Hypothermia is defined as a core body temperature of less than 35°C, with a progression of symptoms visible as the body continues to cool.[28] Core body temperatures between 32°C and 35°C are classified as mild hypothermia and typically show symptoms of confusion, slurred speech, and mild ataxia. Pulse, blood pressure (BP), and respiratory rate is likely to be elevated. Shivering is present at this level of decrease in temperature. Moderate hypothermia is defined as a core temperature between 28°C and 31°C (82.4°F–87.8°F) and shows progressive symptoms, including lethargy. Hallucinations may be present. Pulse, BP, and respiratory rate are lowered, and shivering generally ceases. Cardiac arrhythmias can be seen at this level. Severe hypothermia involves core temperatures of less than 28°C. At this degree of cold injury, spontaneous movement ceases, and pulse and respirations slow. Prolonged severe exposure leads to further bradycardia, spontaneous arrhythmias, and subsequent death.[29]

All patients identified to have a decreased temperature should be aggressively protected from further heat loss. Movement out of a cold environment, removal of wet clothing, and use of blankets are recommended.[30] Quick evaluation of core temperature (rectally) is critical. Of note, many oral and rectal thermometers only register to 35°C; thus for colder events, medical preparation should include acquiring lower range thermometers. As soon as possible, cardiac rhythm should be evaluated. Stability should be assessed, and the pulseless patient should be treated emergently with defibrillation, establishment of a secure airway, warmed oxygen ventilation, and infusion of warmed saline, all in preparation for immediate transport to an emergency medical facility. In patients with moderate to severe hypothermia, care should be taken during manipulation and treatment, because excessive movement may stimulate arrhythmias.[31] In any of the situations described earlier, constant monitoring should be maintained to watch for temperature change, mental status changes, and any progression in symptoms. Effective passive rewarming efforts should result in an average temperature increase of 0.4°C to 2°C per hour.[13]

For collapsed but responsive athletes who are initially normothermic and do not demonstrate a focal evident concern, **Fig. 3** suggests an approach for a consistent evaluation. This group likely comprises the bulk of patients needing care; therefore, the ability to efficiently and effectively triage and treat these athletes is of great importance. The patient should be placed in the supine position, with the legs elevated 12 to 24 inches above the level of the chest. In this situation, an initial assessment of level of consciousness and apparent degree of dehydration should be completed. For patients with an altered level of consciousness, active emesis, or overt signs of dehydration, intravenous access should be pursued quickly and 1 L of normal saline should be administered. If immediate electrolyte testing is available on site, blood should be withdrawn before fluid administration, and sodium and glucose levels should be obtained. Patients should be monitored at close intervals for vital signs, including continued attention to pulse, BP, and rectal temperature as well as any changes to mental status. As long as these patients are showing stability and improvement in symptoms, it may be safe to continue care on site and maintain rehydration as appropriate. If mental status changes are persistent or if vital signs continue to demonstrate abnormalities (pulse >100, systolic BP <110, temperature >40°C), or if significant electrolyte abnormalities can be identified, the patient should be prepared for transport.

The remainder of patients with normothermia, without significant evidence of dehydration, active emesis, or altered mental status, can be effectively treated with continued oral rehydration and rest in a supine position with the legs elevated. Regular reassessment is recommended to evaluate mental status and vital signs. Providers should be mindful of patients demonstrating progressive worsening of initial mild or nonobvious symptoms, and may not manifest significant vital sign or mental status changes until later.[32]

Patients with normothermia who demonstrate altered mental status, persistent nausea/vomiting, or paresthesias should be suspected for exertional hyponatremia. Hypotonic oral fluids should be avoided, because this can worsen progressive hypo-natremia and may impair the ability to create dilute urine. The use of isotonic and hypertonic saline can be considered for more severe cases, but providers should be well aware of the risks and concerns with these therapies.[33] See http://champ. usuhs.mil/chclinicaltools.html for further discussion and recommendations.

According to the discretion of the medical staff, patients should be observed for a period of time that allows reassurance of a stable and improving condition. This confidence may be affected by the presence or absence of friends or family members who can assist with ambulation and observe for future symptomatic changes in improved patients. Runners without specific concerns, who have proved to be stable and have regained the ability to walk under their own power, can generally be released safely. Broad precautions should be given regarding progressive symptoms (ie, mental status changes or seizure in hyponatremia), signs of rhabdomyolysis (wors-ening pain, swelling, and motion difficulties), and end-organ failure (oliguria), along with specific recommendations for any other observed concerns.

OFFICE-BASED MANAGEMENT

Patients who present in a clinical setting after an episode of collapse can present a different set of challenges. While the acuity is certainly diminished, the uncertainty regarding a clear cause may be heightened. Assuming that the patient has recovered adequately to seek further evaluation, a systematic approach can again be helpful, not because of a need to rapidly assess and treat, but to be thorough and effective in assessment and further care. In the setting of a recovered collapse, until there is confi-dence of a particular diagnosis it is important to remember that the runner should be discouraged from further activity during the evaluation.[34] Although this seems like a straightforward recommendation, providers who care for runners understand how difficult it may be to convince these patients of the need for appropriate activity restric-tion during the length of time needed for appropriate evaluation.

The greatest available tool to the provider in this situation is the ability to take a more detailed history. As was alluded to in the previous section, the timing of the event becomes very important when attempting to discern the differential diagnoses. Collapse that occurs after completion of activity is more likely to be associated with orthostatic or postural hypotension, which is discussed in the section on EAC. Collapse occurring before the completion of an event is far more concerning for an underlying cardiac source, including ischemia, arrhythmia, structural defects, and so forth.[35] These are far from exclusive distinctions, but the difference can be helpful in framing subsequent historical questions.

Any information from the patient regarding an evaluation that might have been made at the time of collapse can be helpful. This information could include eyewitness accounts regarding changes in the level of consciousness, and irregular behaviors before and during an episode of collapse. Although it is rarely available, records of care rendered at a mass participation event or from an emergency room visit after episode of collapse would certainly be pertinent. Obviously, there is little ability to retrospectively confirm a diagnosis of acute heat injury, hyponatremia, hyperthermia, or several other diagnoses without a clear record of care from the time of treatment.

Several other historical clues can be helpful. Any presence of prodromal symptoms such as chest pain or palpitations would certainly raise suspicion of a cardiac cause. Abrupt collapse without any associated symptoms may increase suspicion for arrhythmia. Collapse associated with sudden loud noises or rapid temperature changes, such as cold water, might be the result of LQTS. Precedent pruritus or wheezing might indicate a case of exercise-induced anaphylaxis. Postictal symptoms or the loss of bowel or bladder control would be more suggestive of a seizure disorder. Patients with vasovagal presyncope or syncope may report symptoms such as light-headedness, diaphoresis, tunnel vision, or nausea prior to the collapse. The symptoms described earlier, particularly those classically associated with vasovagal syncope, are not exclusive and should not be used to support inaction in a further workup and evaluation. In addition to the event-specific history, the risk for cardiac origin must be further assessed by exploring any pertinent factors such as hypertension, hyperlipidemia, diabetes, smoking, and family history of known heart disease or unexplained deaths.

The physical examination can be directed toward pertinent concerns from the history, but it is prudent to remember that many of the descriptions can be extremely nonspecific, and a broad examination should consistently incorporate certain items. In addition to standard vital signs, BP readings should be obtained from the upper and lower extremities. Pulse and BP readings should be obtained in the supine and standing positions, separated by at least 3 minutes.[36] A dynamic cardiac examination should be completed, involving the auscultation of multiple points with the patient situated in 2 different positions to elicit differing degrees of preload such as squatting and standing, or with Valsalva. A systolic murmur that is increased during standing may be suggestive of obstructive hypertrophic cardiomyopathy. Further cardiac examination should include the presence or absence of thrills and an atypical point of maximal cardiac impulse. Pertinent vascular findings would include carotid bruits and pulse abnormalities such as a brachial femoral delay, bifid pulse, or a slow rising pulse. A full neurologic examination should be performed, with careful attention to any focal motor or sensory deficits and the presence of abnormal or asymmetric reflexes.

Once a detailed history and careful physical are completed, specific laboratory studies may be appropriate. Electrolyte abnormalities might increase suspicion for arrhythmia or underlying metabolic disorder. Likewise, a diminished blood count would be consistent with a symptomatic anemia, which could certainly result in collapse. In using laboratory studies for retrospective evaluation of collapse, it is important to remember that normal laboratory findings should not provide undue reassurance against underlying pathologic conditions. Likewise, the observance of abnormalities in a laboratory evaluation may not preclude the possibility of other underlying pathologic conditions. In short, while laboratory studies may be helpful in further evaluation of collapse in the outpatient setting, it is critical that their use does not discourage further assessment of cardiovascular abnormalities.

It is recommended that the outpatient evaluation of patients who are suspected of syncope or presyncope associated with exercise should include an electrocardiogram.[37] In cases where the history is less consistent with cardiac origin, a normal electrocardiogram (ECG) may provide some reassurance. However, more pertinent are the potential findings that may be associated with underlying pathology that could be associated with syncope or collapse. Clearly, abnormal findings on ECG may allow for more prompt and direct evaluation of certain conditions. **Table 1** lists several conditions that may be seen in ERS with associated abnormal findings on an ECG. Caution is again advised in using findings from an ECG to definitively diagnose certain pathologic conditions or to rule out the possibility of other underlying cardiovascular conditions, because many findings do not correlate strongly with predictable outcome patterns.[38] Two additional factors are important to remember. First, some conditions that are known to be high-risk conditions for ERS, such as coronary artery anomalies,

Table 1
Clinical findings, correlative ECG findings, and recommended evaluation of various conditions associated with collapse

Diagnosis	Clinical Clues	Electrocardiogram	Suggested Diagnostic Testing
Neurocardiogenic syncope	Noxious stimulus, prolonged upright position	Normal	Exercise testing
Supraventricular tachyarrhythmias	Palpitations, response to carotid sinus pressure	Preexcitation	Electrophysiologic study and definitive therapy
Hypertrophic cardiomyopathy	Grade III/VI systolic murmur, louder with Valsalva, when present	Normal; pseudoinfarction pattern; left ventricular hypertrophy with strain	Echocardiography with Doppler
Myocarditis	Prior upper respiratory tract infection, pneumonia; shortness of breath; recreational drug use	Simulating a myocardial infarction with ectopy	Viral studies; echocardiogram; drug screening
Aortic stenosis	Exertional syncope; grade III/VI harsh systolic crescendo-decrescendo murmur	Left ventricular hypertrophy	Echocardiography with Doppler
Mitral valve prolapse	"Thumping heart"; midsystolic click with or without a murmur	QT interval may be prolonged	Echocardiography with Doppler
Prolonged QT syndrome	Recurrent syncope with family history of sudden death	Prolonged corrected QT interval (>44)	Family history; exercise stress test with ECG after exercise
Coronary anomalies	Usually asymptomatic; sudden death event	Normal rest electrocardiogram	Coronary angiography; cardiac MR imaging
Acquired coronary artery diseases	Chest pain syndrome, family history	Ischemia; may be normal	Exercise testing with or without perfusion or contractile imaging
Right ventricular dysplasia	Asymptomatic until syncope; tachyarrhythmias	T wave inversion v1–v3 PVCs with LBBB configuration	Echo/Doppler study; electrocardiography.
EAC: functional sympatholysis	Collapse after finish line; "being out of it," even in the supine position with normal heart rate and BP	Normal	Only as clinically indicated; generally requires reassurance

Abbreviations: LBBB, left bundle branch block; PVC, premature ventricular contraction.

typically show no resting ECG changes.[39] Secondly, some ECG findings that are otherwise associated with pathologic conditions may be considered normal in athletes. Sinus bradycardia, first and second-degree heart block, early repolarization, and voltage criteria for left ventricular hypertrophy are all findings that may be seen normally in the resting ECGs of higher-level athletes.[40]

The variability of findings described in the history and physical, laboratory evaluation, and ECG all underscore the difficulty in the nonacute evaluation of patients after exertional collapse. In cases that are clearly evident after history, physical, ECG, and pertinent laboratory findings, appropriate treatment may be rendered and return to running or other activity can be cautiously directed according to the specific condition. In cases without a clearly identified cause for the collapse, it is recommended that a thorough cardiovascular evaluation be pursued. The included algorithm (**Fig. 4**) suggests a pathway for this evaluation.

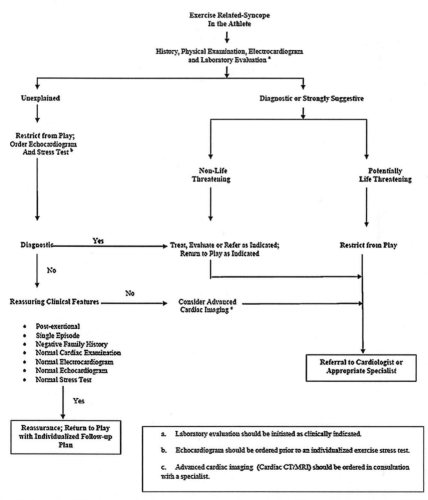

Fig. 4. An algorithmic approach to the evaluation and initial management of ERS in athletes.

FURTHER DIAGNOSTIC TESTING

For cases of collapse that cannot be attributed easily to benign or clearly identified conditions, the remaining evaluation should be completed in a systematic fashion according to the risk and likelihood of associated conditions. In these cases, cardiac concerns remain the highest risk for subsequent mortality. The remainder of the evaluation should be targeted at these various cardiac conditions. Given the increased prevalence of structural cardiac abnormalities, an echocardiograph is strongly recommended. Echocardiograph allows for an evaluation of valvular structure, left and right ventricular size and function, aortic annulus size, and estimated pulmonary artery pressures. In some cases, it may be possible to evaluate the coronary ostia. Because most cases of significant coronary artery anomalies involve a transposition at the level of the ostia, well-visualized, normal-appearing ostia can essentially rule out abnormalities. If echocardiography does not yield an overt diagnosis or there is an increased suspicion of ischemic disease, then stress testing may also play a valuable role. There are a few concerns with stress testing in runners or other athletes. First, unless the evaluation is being directed by a consultant, who is well experienced in the assessment of athletes, the possibility of structural disease should mandate that echocardiography be completed before stress testing. Also, it is likely that typical stress testing protocols (Bruce, Ramp, and so forth) may not induce sufficient stress to elicit a diagnostic finding in runners or other athletes. It may be necessary to construct a higher intensity scenario to create an adequate cardiac demand on the runner.

In situations where echocardiography and stress testing are unfruitful, there are newer imaging techniques that may help further clarify other conditions associated with syncope and collapse. High-resolution computed tomographic angiography (CTA) and cardiac magnetic resonance imaging (MRI) with gadolinium have shown an ability to evaluate several pertinent conditions, such as hypertrophic cardiomyopathy, coronary artery anomalies, myocardial fibrosis, and smaller structural defects.[41] There is a balance between the specific risks and benefits to each of these studies, and these concerns can help direct the appropriate study for each scenario. For example, CTA has shown an improved ability over cardiac MRI to follow the full course of a coronary artery, better identifying deeply tunneled arteries or sharply angled ostia. Despite this advantage, there is some hesitancy in reflexively pursuing CTA because of the substantial radiation exposure. Unless other options are unavailable, CTA should be avoided in younger women because of the increased lifetime risk of breast cancer.[42] The decision regarding the appropriate study depends on the patient and available resources, and should be made in conjunction with a consulting specialist.

Beyond the means discussed earlier, ambulatory monitoring may help further evaluate the possibility of arrhythmia. Depending on the frequency and pattern of suspicious symptoms, the options would include event monitors, Holter monitors, and continuous loop recorders. Holter monitors may be useful in cases of frequent or easily reproducible symptoms. However, the known yield on these devices is relatively low to begin with. In patients who have presenting symptoms only during exercise, the brief period of time captured by Holter monitors may render these devices less helpful.[43] For patients with less frequent or predictable symptoms who have not demonstrated findings on stress testing, longer term electrical monitoring with a continuous loop event recorder can be more appropriate.[44] These devices are designed to provide monitoring over the course of weeks or months, and newer models are designed to be implanted under the skin, negating the need for wearing the device and accompanying electrodes during exercise.

Among the various diagnostic tools available to physicians in cases of collapse or syncope, tilt table testing requires discussion in this context. In cases of collapse during exercise, there may be specific concerns about the limitations of tilt table testing. Tilt table testing does not replicate the stressful environment of exercise, and a negative test would thus offer no insight as to whether the origin of the collapse or syncope is neurally mediated. In addition, because of increased vagal tone that can be seen in runners and other athletes, patients may be greatly susceptible to orthostatic hypotension. This tendency may result in an increased likelihood of a positive result during tilt table testing, and may provide unfounded confidence in a diagnosis that may be coincident, and not the true underlying cause of the collapse.[45] For these reasons, significant caution is advised when considering tilt table testing to further evaluate cases of collapse or syncope associated with exercise.

In the outpatient setting, the challenges of evaluating collapse may seem daunting. The broad differential and the potential for significant underlying pathology can be frustrating, and there is a temptation to make presumptive diagnoses such as vasovagal syncope, dehydration, and exhaustion. The problem lies in the inability to make definitive conclusions in these diagnoses and the potential for overlooking more significant issues. This is the rationale behind the use of a systematic approach such as the one outlined here, in that it allows a consistent and thorough process for evaluating patients after a collapse episode.

CONSULTATION/TREATMENT

The definitive diagnosis and treatment options in the outpatient setting are broad and are ultimately determined by the level of concern after the initial evaluation. Several conditions benefit from a more urgent and expedited evaluation. Examples of concerning factors include syncope during exercise, collapse preceded by chest pain or palpitations, abrupt collapse without any prodromal symptoms, collapse preceded by loud noise or exposure to cold water, and runners with known history of cardiovascular disease or family history of sudden cardiac death. Collapse attributable to seizures, metabolic disorders, and other noncardiac conditions can often be managed according to well-established recommendations and guidelines. Providers should be mindful of the role of consultant specialists, because many of these patients benefit from appropriate comanagement.

For cases where a cardiovascular etiology has been identified, the 36th Bethesda Guidelines offer an extensive and well-established resource for physicians in the appropriate degree of activity restriction and return to play.[46] This document is extremely thorough and goes into significant detail specific to each condition; so it is strongly recommended that these guidelines be consulted once a diagnosis is made. It is equally advisable that these decisions be made in conjunction with a consulting specialist, particularly when navigating pharmacologic treatment, or other therapies such as revascularization or the use of an automatic implantable cardioverter defibrillator.

SUMMARY

Episodes of collapse are not uncommon in runners. The ability to quickly assess and treat runners in the acute setting is critically important, because collapse can represent a wide spectrum of conditions, ranging from sudden cardiac death to postural hypotension. Initial evaluation and treatment attempts are targeted at the most dire conditions. The described algorithms offer a systematic means by which these patients can be triaged quickly, and life-saving treatment can be initiated without unnecessary delay. Although the protocols described in the acute setting can be extremely helpful in avoiding tragic outcomes at the time immediately following collapse, there remains a significant number of patients who survive a collapse event without obvious sequelae and need subsequent outpatient treatment after it can be assured that they are stable. Given the breadth of diagnoses that may manifest in collapse, a systematic approach can be just as important in the outpatient setting, so that critical conditions are not overlooked and unhelpful studies can be avoided.

For a specific population such as runners, collapse is a challenging situation. Whether assessing many patients in a mass participation event or a single patient in a clinical setting, the value of a well thought-out approach can be the key to successful management. Whether in the discovery and avoidance of life-threatening conditions or the safe and confident return to activity for benign conditions, a thorough pattern of evaluation and treatment can meet the challenge of this difficult diagnosis.

REFERENCES

1. Maron BJ, Shirani J, Poliac LC, et al. Sudden death in young competitive athletes. Clinical, demographic, and pathological profiles. JAMA 1996;276(3):199–204.
2. Campbell R. Runner dies during Marine Corps Marathon. Special to. The Washington Post; 2006. [Online].
3. Associated Press. 3 dead Detroit marathoners said to be healthy. 2009. [Online].
4. Roberts WO. Exercise-associated collapse in endurance events. A classification system. Phys Sportsmed 1989;17:49–57.
5. Driscoll DJ, Jacobsen SJ, Porter CJ, et al. Syncope in children and adolescents. J Am Coll Cardiol 1997;29(5):1039–45.
6. Amital H, Glikson M, Burstein M. Clinical characteristics of unexpected death among young enlisted military personnel: results of a three-decade retrospective surveillance. Chest 2004;126(2):528–33.
7. Colivicchi F, Ammirati F, Santini M. Epidemiology and prognostic implications of syncope in young competing athletes. Eur Heart J 2004;25(19):1749–53.
8. Hobbs JB, Peterson DR, Moss AJ, et al. Risk of aborted cardiac arrest or sudden cardiac death during adolescence in the long-QT syndrome. JAMA 2006;296(10): 1249–54.
9. Corrado D, Basso C, Fontaine G, et al. Clinical profile of young competitive athletes who died suddenly of arrhythmogenic right ventricular cardiomyopathy/dysplasia: a multicenter study. Pacing Clin Electrophysiol 2002;25:544.
10. Holtzhausen L, Noakes TD, Kroning B, et al. Clinical and biochemical characteristics of collapsed ultramarathon runners. Med Sci Sports Exerc 1994;26: 1095–101.
11. Hiller WD, O'Toole ML, Fortess EE, et al. Medical and physiological considerations in triathlons. Am J Sports Med 1987;15(2):164–8.
12. Laird RH. Medical care at ultraendurance triathlons. Med Sci Sports Exerc 1989; 21(5):S222–5.
13. Roberts WO. A 12-yr profile of medical injury and illness for the Twin Cities Marathon. Med Sci Sports Exerc 2000;32(9):1549–55.
14. Roberts WO. Heat and cold: what does the environment do to marathon injury? Sports Med 2007;37(4–5):400–3.
15. O'Connor FG, Bunt CW, Switaj TL. Collapse in a mass participation event: a descriptive study. Clin J Sport Med 2006;16(5):434.

16. Maron BJ, Poliac LC, Roberts WO. Risk for sudden cardiac death associated with marathon running. J Am Coll Cardiol 1996;28:428–31.

17. Roberts WO, Maron BJ. Evidence for decreasing occurrence of sudden cardiac death associated with the marathon. J Am Coll Cardiol 2005;46:1373–4.

18. Levine BD, Buckley JC, Fritsch JM, et al. Physical fitness and cardiovascular regulation: mechanisms of orthostatic intolerance. J Appl Physiol 1991;70:112–22.

19. Smith ML, Graitzer HM, Hudson DL, et al. Baroreflex function in endurance- and static-exercise trained men. J Appl Physiol 1988;64:585–91.

20. Luft UC, Myrhe LG, Leopsky JA, et al. A study of factors affecting tolerance of gravitational stress simulated by lower body negative pressure. Research Report on Specialized Physiology Studies in Support of Manned Space Flight. Contract NAS9-14472. Albuquerque (NM): Lovelace Foundation; 1976. p. 2–60.

21. Available at: http://champ.usuhs.mil/chclinicaltools.html. Accessed November 12, 2009.

22. O'Connor FG, Brennan F, Adirim T, et al. Managing exercise-associated collapse in endurance events. Am J Med Sports 2003;5(3):212–8.

23. Casa DJ, Becker SM, Ganio MS, et al. Validity of devices that assess body temperature during outdoor exercise in the heat. J Athl Train 2007;42(3):333–42.

24. Ronneberg K, Roberts WO, McBean AD, et al. Temporal artery temperature measurements do not detect hyperthermic marathon runners. Med Sci Sports Exerc 2008;40(8):1373–5.

25. Howe AS, Boden BP. Heat-related illness in athletes. Am J Sports Med 2007; 35(8):1384–95.

26. McDermott BP, Casa DJ, Ganio MS, et al. Acute whole-body cooling for exercise-induced hyperthermia: a systematic review. J Athl Train 2009;44(1):84–93.

27. Taylor NA, Caldwell JN, Van den Heuvel AM, et al. To cool, but not too cool: that is the question—immersion cooling for hyperthermia. Med Sci Sports Exerc 2008; 40(11):1962–9.

28. Pozos RS, Danzl DF. Human physiological responses to cold stress and hypothermia. In: Pandolf KB, Burr RE, editors. Textbooks of military medicine: medical aspects of harsh environments, vol. 1. Falls Church (VA): Office of the Surgeon General, U.S. Army; 2002. p. 351–82.

29. Graham CA, McNaughton GW, Wyatt JP. The electrocardiogram in hypothermia. Wilderness Environ Med 2001;12(4):232–5.

30. Biem J, Koehncke N, Classen D, et al. Out of the cold: management of hypothermia and frostbite. CMAJ 2003;168(3):305–11.

31. Nielsen HK, Toft P, Koch J, et al. Hypothermic patients admitted to an intensive care unit: a fifteen year survey. Dan Med Bull 1992;39(2):190–3.

32. Goudie AM, Tunstall-Pedoe DS, Kerins M, et al. Exercise-associated hyponatraemia after a marathon: case series. J R Soc Med 2006;99(7):363–7.

33. Rosner MH, Kirven J. Exercise-associated hyponatremia. Clin J Am Soc Nephrol 2007;2(1):151–61.

34. O'Connor FG, Oriscello RG, Levine BD. Exercise-related syncope in the young athlete: reassurance, restriction or referral? Am Fam Physician 1999;60(7):2001–8.

35. Link M, Estes NA. How to manage athletes with syncope. Cardiology Clin 2007; 25(3):457–66.

36. Kapoor WN. Current evaluation and management of syncope. Circulation 2002; 106(13):1606–9.

37. Maron BJ, Thompson PD, Ackerman MJ, et al. Recommendations and considerations related to preparticipation screening for cardiovascular abnormalities in competitive athletes: 2007 update. Circulation 2007;115:1643–55.

38. Pelliccia A, Di Paolo FM, Quattrini FM, et al. Outcomes in athletes with marked ECG repolarization abnormalities. N Engl J Med 2008;358(2):152–61.
39. Lawless CE, Best TM. Electrocardiograms in athletes: interpretation and diagnostic accuracy. Med Sci Sports Exerc 2008;40(5):787–98.
40. Zehender M, Meinertz T, Keul J, et al. ECG variants and cardiac arrhythmias in athletes: clinical relevance and prognostic importance. Am Heart J 1990;119: 1378–91.
41. Crean A. Cardiovascular MR and CT in congenital heart disease. Heart 2007; 93(12):1637–47.
42. Hurwitz LM, Reiman RE, Yoshizumi TT. Radiation dose from contemporary cardiothoracic multidetector CT protocols with an anthropomorphic female phantom: implications for cancer induction. Radiology 2007;245(3):742–50.
43. Krahn AD, Klein GJ, Yee R, et al. Use of an extended monitoring strategy in patients with problematic syncope. Circulation 1999;99:406–10.
44. Paisey JR, Yue AM, Treacher K, et al. Implantable loop recorders detect tachyarrhythmias in symptomatic patients with negative electrophysiological studies. Int J Cardiol 2005;98(1):35–8.
45. Kosinski D, Grubb BP, Karas BJ, et al. Exercise-induced neurocardiogenic syncope: clinical data, pathophysiological aspects, and potential role of tilt table testing. Europace 2000;2(1):77–82.
46. Maron BJ, Zipes DP. 36th Bethesda Conference: eligibility recommendations for competitive athletes with cardiovascular abnormalities. J Am Coll Cardiol 2005; 45:2–64.

The Female Runner: Gender Specifics

Stacy L. Lynch, MD, Anne Z. Hoch, DO*

KEYWORDS

• Female runner • Gender specifics • Female athlete triad
• Exercise and pregnancy • Stress incontinence

The magnitude of benefits that exercise has on the health and well-being of female athletes is continually being expanded. Before trailblazers such as Babe Didrikson Zaharias, women were not included in most athletic endeavors. Relegated to the sidelines, women had to wait their turn on the playing field. The face of athletics changed dramatically in 1972 with the passage of the Title IX of the Education Amendments, which specifically prohibited sex discrimination in education and programs that receive federal funding[1]:

> No person in the United States shall, on the basis of sex, be excluded from participation in, be denied the benefits of, or be subjected to discrimination under any education program or activity receiving federal financial assistance.

Since Title IX was enacted, female participation in sports has sky-rocketed. Women's participation in Division I college athletics rose from a mere 15% in 1971 to 44% in 2004. In 1972, 1 in 27 girls played high school sports or 7%; today, almost half (41%) of high school girls play, an increase of more than 1000%.[2] The applaudable efforts of Title IX have resulted in athletics opportunities for 2.9 million high school girls and more than 170,000 collegiate women in 2006–2007 with 21,516 college women participating in outdoor track and field.[3]

In the past 35 years, girls and women stopped being just spectators and cheerleaders, and became players. This changed far more than just their after-school activities; it increased their self-esteem, reduced risky behaviors such as drug use and teen pregnancy, and gave them life skills.[4] Mariah Burton Nelson wrote "Sport for women represents autonomy, strength, pleasure, community, control, justice and power …. It changes everything."[5] Today, an overwhelming number of female athletes compete recreationally, competitively, and professionally. Images of the female athlete appear on the covers of magazines and posters on bedroom walls. Young women today are

---

There was no funding needed to support this work.
Department of Orthopaedic Surgery, Sports Medicine Center, Medical College of Wisconsin, 8700 Watertown Plank Road, Milwaukee, WI 53226, USA
* Corresponding author.
E-mail address: azeni@mcw.edu

Clin Sports Med 29 (2010) 477–498
doi:10.1016/j.csm.2010.03.003
0278-5919/10/$ – see front matter © 2010 Elsevier Inc. All rights reserved.

presented with female role models from a variety of sports ranging from tennis and golf to track and field. The legacy of Title IX will be the generations of inspirational stories of female athletes that made a difference in their sport, community, and world. However, it is evident that girls who live in the suburbs have benefited much more than urban dwellers. Only 36% of city girls describe themselves as "moderately active" compared with 50% of girls who live in suburbs according to a 2007 survey.[6]

The 1928 Olympics in Amsterdam ushered in a new era of female athletics. For the first time, women were allowed to compete in track and field events. Although inclusion of women was a milestone, the longest race sanctioned by the International Olympic Committee for the next 32 years was the 200 m. In 1960, women were given the opportunity to compete in the 800 m followed by the inclusion of 1500 m in 1972. The 23rd Olympiad in 1984 included the running of the first Olympic woman's marathon. In the 2000 Sydney games, the Olympic distance triathlon was introduced for men and women. Female athletes have come a long way. Only 36 women competed in the 1908 Olympics blazing a trail for the 4746 female athletes that ran, jumped, and played in the 2008 games. In these most recent games (Beijing, China, 2008) more than 42% of Olympic athletes were female.[7] With greater involvement and increased notoriety, female involvement in athletics is continuing to make strides toward equality. Specifically for the United States, 52% (N = 310) of athletes were men and 48% (N = 286) were women.[8] The US track and field team consisted of 59 women[9] and 74 men.[10] Overall, the United States won 110 medals; the men's track and field team won 14 medals and the women's track and field team won 9.[11]

Women are now integral in the sports entertainment industry and endorsements of female athletic superstars rival those of their male counterparts. You can now turn on your television and watch women in sports from the Women's Soccer World Cup to the Women's National Basketball Association (WNBA) to the Ladies Professional Golf Association (LPGA). In 2000, US$25 billion was generated through merchandise associated with female sports attire. The athletic shoe and apparel industry anticipates this amount to top $38 billion throughout the decade.[12] The Williams sisters alone have endorsed millions of dollars, Serena making US$14 million with endorsements including Hewlett-Packard, Nike, and Kraft, and Venus making US$13 million in earnings.[13]

With an increase in visibility and a greater acceptance of female athletics, women of all ages are turning to sports for recreation, health and fitness, weight management, social interaction, competition, and personal accomplishment. Running is an integral component of most training regimens. Regardless of motivation for running, long or short distances, it is essential that the effect that running may have on the overall wellness of female athletes is understood. This article outlines the anatomic, physiologic, and psychological issues of the female runner. The updated female athlete triad position stand is discussed as well as new research showing that athletic amenorrhea is associated with increased cardiovascular risk.

GENDER DIFFERENCES

There are significant physiologic, anatomic, and psychological issues facing the female runner compared with their male counterparts. Risk factors for running injuries in women are divided into 2 categories: extrinsic (training surface, shoes, and orthotic equipment) and intrinsic (age, sex, phase of the menstrual cycle, biomechanics, and fitness levels).[14] This section focuses on some of the intrinsic factors that affect the female runner. A thorough understanding of these unique factors is essential for comprehensive care of the female runner.

Prepubescent Body

Before puberty, there are no significant differences between boys and girls with regard to body composition and biomechanics. Before puberty, boys and girls have similar height, weight, muscle mass, heart size, sports performance, and aerobic capabilities.[15] According to Hewett and colleagues,[16] male and female athletes have similar forces and motions about the knee when they land from a jump before maturation. However, after puberty, neuromuscular control of the knee changes significantly for women.[16] Girls enter puberty earlier than boys. Preceding sexual maturation, the female adolescent peek growth spurt occurs at approximately 11.8 years of age compared with 13.4 years in the adolescent male.[17] The principal gender differences in body composition and mechanics become apparent during puberty as a result of sex hormones.

Body Composition

Unlike the prepubertal runner, the body compensation of postpubertal male and female runners is very different. Men and women produce exactly the same hormones, just in different ratios. Androgens, produced in the female adrenal glands and ovaries (testicles in men), are the hormones that influence total muscle mass and therefore strength. Testosterone and androstenedione are the most important androgens for strength development. Women, on average, produce approximately one-seventh of the testosterone that men produce; however, this small quantity of testosterone is still essential for normal sexual development and maintenance of emotional and physical health.[18] The total cross-sectional area of muscle in the adult woman is 60% compared with 80% in the adult man.[19] As a result, maximal strength measures and maximal power measures may be reduced in women. When a strength/lean body mass ratio is controlled for, women and men are almost equal in strength, and when strength is calculated from the cross-sectional area of muscle, no significant gender difference exists.[20] If the quality of muscle is not different between men and women, then it seems that the strength and power differences between the sexes are likely a function of muscle quantity rather than quality.[21] Although hormones play a role in strength development, it is unclear whether they are the reason for the differences in absolute strength.[20]

Estrogen is another hormone responsible for the differences between male and female athletes. The percentage of body fat differs between men and women. Adult women usually have 22% to 26% body fat and men have 13% to 16%.[22,23] Estrogen is responsible for greater amounts of fat weight in women and testosterone is responsible for greater lean body weight in men. Elite female runners have larger body fat reserves compared with male runners. As stated by Noakes[24] in 1991, elite female runners carry approximately 5 kg more body fat and about 3 kg less lean mass than male runners.[24] With an increased percentage of body fat, female athletes are more buoyant and better insulated.[25]

Healthy Bones

Athletes have higher bone mineral density (BMD) than sedentary premenopausal women.[26,27] It seems that the largest increases in BMD in female athletes occur when impact sports are started 5 years before menarche.[28] In addition, sports with a high amount of "irregular weight bearing" have been shown to increase BMD to a greater degree in men and women.[29] In childhood, bone mass accrual occurs through growth in length, width, and accumulation of bone minerals. A significant increase in BMD occurs with pubertal growth. At age 12 years, young girls have

83% of their total body BMD. Two years after menarche, 95% of their BMD has formed.[30] Bone growth in girls ceases approximately at age 20 years. In boys, bone growth continues until the early 20s.[31] The effects of estrogen on BMD is discussed in more detail later in this article.

Physiologically

Sex hormones not only influence body composition; they also have a large impact on the respiratory and cardiovascular systems. Female athletes have smaller heart size, smaller heart volume, and lower diastolic pressure than male athletes, even when controlled for body weight.[22] With a heart smaller in size and volume, women naturally have a smaller stroke volume. Based on the equation: cardiac output = stroke volume × heart rate, women also have an increased heart rate for a given submaximal cardiac output.[25,32,33] Even with an increased heart rate, a female athlete's cardiac output is approximately 30% lower than an equally trained male's cardiac output because of the lower stroke volume found in women.[25] A female athlete's systolic blood pressure is also lower than her male counterparts.[32] In addition to the cardiac differences, men have approximately 6% more red blood cells and 10% to 15% more hemoglobin per 100 mL of blood than women, increasing the oxygen-carrying capacity of male athletes.[34,35] With a larger absolute heart size and a greater total blood volume, the male cardiovascular system can supply more blood per minute to working muscles. In addition to having lower cardiac output and lower hemoglobin level, women also have a lower vital capacity when controlled for body weight. Female athletes also have smaller lungs.[22]

Combining the differences between men and women in the cardiac and pulmonary systems, the difference in the total oxygen-carrying capacity is amplified. Vo_{2max} is 15% to 25% lower in women even after controlling for the differences in body weight and percentage of body fat.[25] Recent evidence also suggests that during heavy aerobic exercise, women have greater expiratory flow limitations, increased work of breathing, and possibly greater exercise-induced arterial hypoxemia than men.[36] In the 1980s, Cureton and colleagues[37,38] reported that the weight issue from the higher percent body fat and the reduced red cell count accounted for at least part of the differences in running performances between male and female runners. Compared with male endurance athletes, a smaller-framed female with disproportionately smaller pulmonary and cardiovascular systems has a reduced physiologic oxygen delivery system and therefore a performance disadvantage.

Biomechanically

There are numerous anatomic differences unique to the female athlete that ultimately affect running biomechanics.[39] Studies have routinely shown that women run, land, and jump differently from men when playing sports.[40,41] Proprioception and reaction time, postural stability, limb dominance, muscle stiffness, firing patterns, and landing biomechanics are all continually being studied in women.[42] Compared with their male counterparts, adult women tend to be shorter, weigh less, have shorter limbs, and have smaller articular surfaces.[22] These anatomic differences account for less power for striking, kicking, throwing, and running.[43,44] Women have shorter and smaller limbs relative to body length; the length of the lower extremities in women comprises 51.2% of total height compared with 56% in men.[32] Although women tend to have a lower center of gravity, which may provide better balance,[32,43] the center of gravity differences between men and women are minimal and depend more on height and body type than gender.[45]

The alignment pattern of the lower extremities is crucial for female runners who rely on precise biomechanics for optimal performance.[39] In general, women have a wider pelvis but narrower shoulders than men.[32,46] The wider shape of the female pelvis is the foundation of the lower extremity alignment differences between the sexes. Because of the shape of the pelvis, women have increased femoral anteversion and genu valgum. The biomechanical problems female runners face is magnified by hypoplastic vastus medialis obliquus muscle and weak hip abductor muscles. Inadequate hip stabilization may play a role in running-related injuries in women. Ireland and colleagues[47] found that women with patellofemoral pain syndrome had 26% less hip abductor strength and 36% less hip external rotator strength compared with controls without patellofemoral pain.

Ferber and colleagues[48] compared differences in kinematic and kinetic patterns of the hip and knee in 20 male and female recreational runners. Women were found to have significantly greater peak hip adduction angle and hip frontal plane negative work, which may be the result of a greater pelvis width and femoral length ratio in women.[49]

Fredericson and colleagues[50] reported the importance of hip abduction strength in patients with iliotibial band syndrome. After a 6-week hip abduction strengthening program, 22 out of 24 runners experienced a significant decrease in pain and a 35% to 51% increase in hip abduction strength. In a study of 19 young women with patellofemoral pain, Earl and colleagues[51] showed that an 8-week supervised physical therapy program focused on increasing hip abduction, external rotation, and core strength resulted in decreased knee pain and increased functional ability. These results suggest that a hip abduction strengthening program can be effective at preventing and treating running-related injuries in women. Another study by Landry and colleagues[52] found that there are also gastrocnemii differences between elite male and female soccer players such that female players have greater lateral gastrocnemius activity and a mediolateral gastrocnemii imbalance that was not present in male players.

Psychologically

Psychological factors are of particular importance to the female runner. In the past several decades the focus on thin, equating to beautiful, has resulted in significant pathology for women in Western cultures. The media bombards the youth of today idealizing thinness and directly affecting the way girls think about their own developing bodies. A study by Davidson and colleagues,[53] which examined the body-shape preferences of children in the United States, China, and Turkey, found that the children from the United States ranked being slim as their top choice. Young women and girls are highly influenced by sociocultural factors relating to body image and eating habits, which strongly correlate with self-image.[54] Even girls who are at a medically healthy weight desire to be thinner[55] for reasons such as peer teasing, parental pressure, feeling uncomfortable or embarrassed, wanting to feel better or look better, changing sports ability, not liking current weight, and wanting to be healthier.[56] The demands on a female athlete to "win at all costs" along with an exceedingly controlling parent or coach, and intensive involvement in sports causing social isolation may increase the athlete's risk for developing particular problems such as disordered eating or an eating disorder.[57] These characteristics are known to be contributing factors in the development of eating disorders as some female athletes attempt to preserve their prepubescent body shape with caloric restriction and radical dieting techniques.

PREGNANCY AND RUNNING

Pregnancy is an additional concern for the female runner. In a survey of American women, 42% exercised during pregnancy, half of whom exercised for longer than 6 months.[58] With so many women running and competing in a variety of sports, it is understandable that they wish to continue their regime during pregnancy. There are benefits to women who voluntarily maintain their exercise regimen during pregnancy including less weight gain (3.4 vs 9.9 kg), less fat deposits (2.2 vs 6.7 kg), increased fitness, lower cardiovascular risk profile, and higher self-assessed body image than those who stop exercising.[59] Exercise during pregnancy also improves mood and physical symptoms such as nausea.[60] Pregnancy also has associated biomechanical changes secondary to weight gain, change in center of gravity and ligament relaxation, all of which may detract from the ability to attain peak performances.[61] In addition, pregnancy is associated with increased requirements for dietary energy, specifically an additional 300 kcal/d is required after the first trimester.[62] In well-nourished women who maintain their activity level during pregnancy (until gestational week 32), the increase in basal metabolic rate represents most of the pregnancy-induced increase in total energy expenditure.[62]

In the absence of either medical or obstetric complications, the American College of Obstetricians and Gynecologists recommends that pregnant women should exercise at least 30 minutes a day on most, if not all days of the week, at an intensity of 60% to 90% of maximal heart rate or 50% to 85% of either maximal oxygen uptake or heart rate reserve as is recommended for healthy nonpregnant women.[63] In addition to avoiding the supine position and exercises that have potential for abdominal trauma, pregnant women should monitor hydration status and body temperature (<38.7°C), stopping exercise for extreme shortness of breath, dizziness, headache, chest pain, or contractions, and should not exercise when fatigued and until exhaustion.[63]

Some elite athletes have trained daily and rigorously until close to delivery without adverse consequences to themselves or their unborn child[64]; however, caution should be used in other female populations. Exercise enhances fetoplacental growth[65] and the placentae of pregnant runners.[66] When comparing women who exercised during pregnancy to nonexercisers, there were no differences in duration of labor, birth weight, or 1- and 5-minute Apgar scores.[67] Women who exercise at high volumes in mid and late pregnancy had significantly lighter (3.39 kg vs 3.81 kg) and thinner (8.3% fat vs 12.1% fat) babies than those babies born of women who reduced their exercise.[65] When looking past initial labor and delivery, the babies of exercising mothers have normal growth and development during the first year of life.[68]

According to the American College of Obstetricians and Gynecologists, there are absolute and relative contraindications to exercise for the pregnant runner.[63] Absolute contraindications include a pregnant woman who has hemodynamically significant heart disease, restrictive lung disease, multiple gestations at risk for premature labor, persistent second or third trimester bleeding, placenta previa after 26 weeks's gestation, premature labor, ruptured membranes, or pregnancy-induced hypertension.[63] Relative contraindications to exercise during pregnancy include women who are severely anemic, morbidly obese, extremely underweight, heavy smokers or have cardiac arrhythmias, chronic bronchitis, poorly controlled diabetes, a history of extremely sedentary lifestyle, intrauterine growth restriction, preeclampsia, orthopedic limitations, poorly controlled seizure disorder, or poorly controlled thyroid disease.[63]

In addition to concerns for pregnant women, there are postpartum concerns. The pregnancy-associated physiologic changes such as ligament relaxation, change in posture, and increased weight[61] may last 4 to 6 weeks postpartum,[63] or longer in women who breast feed. Even though female runners may reduce their training intensity during pregnancy, this does not seem to have a significant effect on their postpartum performance.[69] With the altered or reduced training that occurs during pregnancy, a gradual increase in activity is advised. Compared with nonpregnant women, pregnant women who exercised during pregnancy had a significant increase in absolute Vo_{2max} that was evident 12 to 20 weeks postpartum and was still maintained at 36 to 44 weeks postpartum, as a result of the increased blood volume that occurred during pregnancy.[70] Physical activity can be resumed as soon as physically and medically safe and varies between runners, with some being capable of engaging in an exercise routine within days of delivery.[63] In addition, it is recommended that nursing mothers breast feed before activity to decrease the discomfort caused by breast engorgement and to limit the acidity of milk caused by increased levels of lactic acid.[71]

URINARY INCONTINENCE AND RUNNING

Urinary incontinence (UI) is a frequent complaint of women, and more so in female runners. Bladder symptoms affect women of all ages, however, they are most prevalent among older women.[72] Up to 35% of the total population more than 60 years of age is estimated to be incontinent, with women twice as likely as men to experience incontinence. One in 3 women more than 60 years old have bladder control problems.[73] Stress urinary incontinence (SUI) is involuntary leakage of urine with effort, exertion, or increased abdominal pressures. SUI is common in women of all ages[74] and specific risk factors include female gender, increasing age, multiple vaginal deliveries, postmenopausal status, chronic pelvic pain, obesity, lack of exercise, constipation, and hypertension.[75] In women, there are physical changes resulting from pregnancy, childbirth, and menopause that often contribute to SUI. In female high-level athletes, effort incontinence occurs in all sports involving abrupt repeated increases in intra-abdominal pressure that exceed perineal floor resistance[76] such as high-impact sports activities.[77] The involuntary loss of urine during exercise is often underreported in female athletes which likely is the result of the social implications and embarrassment associated with SUI and lack of awareness of the topic. One study found that more than 90% of those surveyed with SUI had never told anyone about their symptoms.[78] The highest prevalence is found in sports involving high-impact activities such as track and field.[74] In a study of competitive varsity track athletes, Nygaard and colleagues[79] showed that the prevalence of UI while practicing or competing was 26%. Another study by Nygaard[80] found that 35% of Olympian track and field participants had urinary leakage while competing in the Olympic Games. In addition, a study of female elite athletes, aged 15 to 39 years, found the overall SUI prevalence was 41% in these athletes compared with 39% of age-matched controls.[74] SUI is not just a phenomenon of aging women; it also occurs in adolescent runners. More than 25% of high school and college women, aged 14 to 21 years, who completed a survey had symptoms of SUI and/or urge UI while participating in high-impact sports.[78] Unfortunately, more than 90% of those young women with SUI had never told anyone about their UI symptoms.[78] In this same survey, more than 15% of responders with UI reported a "negative effect on their quality of life, impacting their social life or desire to continue participating in sports."[78]

Treatment options for SUI range from more conservative approaches, including behavioral techniques and physical therapy to more aggressive options such as surgery. Behavioral techniques and lifestyle changes include fluid and diet management, planned bathroom trips, and use of pads or protective garments. Physical therapy can be particularly helpful to strengthen the pelvic floor muscles and may incorporate Kegels and electrical stimulation. Medications including anticholinergics, topical estrogen, and imipramine, as well as medical devices like urethral inserts or pessaries, may help control SUI symptoms. More aggressive interventions include interventional therapies (radiofrequency therapy and bulking material injections) and surgery (artificial urinary sphincter, sling procedures, and bladder neck suspension).[81]

OSTEOARTHRITIS AND RUNNING

Runners of advancing age may have arthritic conditions. Osteoarthritis (OA) is the most common form of arthritis in the United States affecting nearly 27 million Americans and resulting in significant joint pain and disability.[82] After the age of 50 years, women are more often affected by OA than men.[83] Although the cause of OA is still unknown, there are risk factors for developing OA such as heredity factors, overweight, joint injury, repeated overuse of certain joints, lack of physical activity, nerve injury, and aging.[84] There have been no studies to date that show a correlation between long-distance running and knee osteoarthritis. Moderate- to high-intensity recreational physical activity has many health benefits and does not result in an increased risk of developing OA.[85] Physical activity, including running, keeps joints flexible and maintains or improves muscle strength, which helps to support the knees and reduce OA symptoms. In addition, losing as few as 5 kg can cut the risk of developing knee OA by 50% for some women.[86] For women with OA, running may be a good form of exercise even if modifications need to be made such as running on softer surfaces or in deep water for symptom control.

THE FEMALE ATHLETE TRIAD: UPDATE

First defined in 1992, the female athlete triad consisted of disordered eating, amenorrhea, and osteoporosis. Since then, there has been a plethora of research in this area. Therefore, the American College of Sports Medicine (ACSM) redefined the female athlete triad in 2007[87] as a spectrum of low energy availability (with or without eating disorders), amenorrhea, and osteoporosis.[87] Each clinical condition is now understood to comprise the pathologic end of a spectrum of interrelated subclinical conditions between health and disease.[87] These components each pose significant health risks to female runners and need to be addressed to maximize prevention, early diagnosis, and treatment.[87]

Disordered Eating

Women who participate in endurance sports, such as running, are at high risk of developing disordered eating, which is a critical component of the female athlete triad. When the ACSM redefined the female athlete triad in 2007, the "disordered eating" category changed to became a "spectrum" ranging from optimal energy availability to low energy availability with or without an eating disorder.[87] As there is a spectrum of energy availability, there is also a spectrum of disordered eating that may range from inadvertent calorie restriction to anorexia nervosa or bulimia nervosa. Energy availability is calculated using dietary energy intake minus exercise energy expenditure and can be expressed as kilocalories/kilogram/lean body mass.[87] It may be low secondary to increased total output (ie, increasing exercise) or by reduced total energy intake (ie, calorie restricting, fasting, binge eating and purging, or use of diet pills and laxatives)[87,88] or a combination of both. Energy availability is the amount of energy remaining for all other bodily functions such as cellular maintenance, thermoregulation, growth, and reproduction.[89] An athlete can still be at a stable body weight while energy availability is low by compensatory mechanisms to restore energy balance (ie, reduced metabolism, decreased energy for reproduction, and cellular maintenance).[87,90,91] A female runner who has increased lean tissue mass may seem to have an adequate weight, however, may not be consuming enough calories to meet her energy needs, which ultimately can lead to menstrual dysfunction, reduced BMD, and decreased performance.

Menstrual Dysfunction

Functional hypothalmic amenorrhea is the second component of the female athlete triad and is a common occurrence amongst female runners. In 2007, the ACSM Position Stand broadened the previous term amenorrhea to include a spectrum of menstrual irregularities ranging from anovulatory eumenorrhea to amenorrhea.[87] There are 2 types of amenorrhea: primary (menstruation cycles not starting by age 15 years) and secondary (the absence of 3 consecutive menstrual periods).[92] Athletic-associated amenorrhea is a complex multifactorial condition that can have grave consequences for young runners. Although physical and emotional stress associated with exercise and competition, percentage of body fat, and genetics can contribute to amenorrhea, low energy availability is the likely predisposing factor. Alterations in resting energy expenditure and metabolic hormones (energy conservation) are increasingly evident across the spectrum of menstrual irregularities including luteal-phase defects, anovulation, and amenorrhea in exercising women.[93] Low energy availability results in endocrine and metabolic changes often leading to hypothalamic-induced athletic amenorrhea,[94] often referred to as functional hypothalamic amenorrhea (FHA), which is the most prevalent cause of amenorrhea in the adolescent age group.[95] There can also be significant changes in allopregnanolone, neuropeptide Y, corticotropin-releasing hormone, leptin, ghrelin, and β-endorphin in women with FHA.[96]

Low BMD

Disordered eating and menstrual irregularities with estrogen deficiency predispose women to the third component of the female athlete triad, osteoporosis.[97] In 2007, the ACSM Position Stand expanded the female athlete triad definition to include a spectrum ranging from optimal bone health to osteoporosis.[87] In 2007, the ACSM also defined the term low BMD as a Z-score between -1.0 and -1.9 and osteoporosis as a Z-score less than or equal to -2.0 with secondary risk factors such as chronic malnutrition, eating disorders, hypogonadism, amenorrhea glucocorticoid exposure, and previous fracture.[87] Osteoporosis does not occur instantaneously with the onset of amenorrhea; however, there is a direct correlation between length of athletic amenorrhea and reduction in BMD.[98] Although genetics determine 60% to 80% of peak bone mass, lifestyle choices including diet (energy availability, calcium, and vitamin D) and physical activity (athletes have a 5%–15% higher BMD than nonathletes[99,100]) are also predictors of bone accrual during growth.[101] This is especially crucial during the female's adolescent growth years because more than one-fourth of adult bone mass is acquired between the ages of 12 and 14 years.[101] A study by Ihle and Loucks[102] found that the rate of bone resorption increased and the rate of bone formation declined within 5 days after energy availability was reduced to less than 30 kcal/kg fat-free mass/d in exercising women. Estrogen is important in regulation of BMD because it limits bone resorption, stimulates calcitonin, and promotes renal retention of calcium.[103] When energy availability is low enough to suppress estrogen, resorption is increased and bone formation is suppressed in dose-response relationships similar to those of insulin, triiodothyronine, and insulinlike growth factor-1.[102]

Prevalence

The female athlete triad or any of its components are prevalent among our youth. A significant number of high school athletes (78%) have 1 or more components of the female athlete triad.[27] A study looking at the prevalence of female athlete triad characteristics in a club triathlon team found that 60% of the triathletes were in a calorie deficit.[104] Another study of 300 female cross-country runners found 19.4% of the runners had previous or current eating disorders.[105] Yet, another study of more than 300 women between the ages of 13 and 39 years found that more elite athletes in leanness sports (46.7%) had clinical eating disorders than athletes in nonleanness sports (19.8%) and controls (21.4%) ($P<.001$).[106]

Amenorrhea is of great concern for runners as it puts them at increased risk for reduced BMD and stress fractures. The prevalence of athletic-associated amenorrhea has been reported to be as high as 60% to 66%, with runners having the highest prevalence.[107] Other studies found that 20% of casual runners and 50% of elite runners report irregular menses.[15] Nichols and colleagues[108] found that 23.5% of high school athletes had evidence of amenorrhea or oligomenorrhea. Hoch and colleagues[27] found a much higher prevalence of 53% in this population, but also found that 21% of sedentary high school students had evidence of menstrual dysfunction.

Given the high prevalence of disordered eating and amenorrhea in women runners, it is not surprising that they have a high prevalence of low BMD. Wiksten-Almstromer and colleagues[109] evaluated the long-term effects on BMD in women diagnosed with menstrual disorders in their adolescence and demonstrated a high frequency of osteopenia/osteoporosis (52%) in adulthood; the strongest predictor of low BMD being a restrictive eating pattern in adolescence. In 2006, Beals and Hill[110] reported 10% of US college athletes from a variety of sports had low BMD defined as Z-scores of −1.0 and −1.9. In high school athletes, Hoch and colleagues[27] and Nichols and colleagues[108] found similar degrees of low BMD Z-scores (−1.0 and −1.9) in 16% and 21.8%.

Studies of high school, college, and elite European athletes have reported the prevalence of simultaneously having all 3 components of the triad to be low. Hoch and colleagues[27] and Nichols and colleagues[108] reported similar findings in high school athletes of 1% and 1.2%, respectively. Beals and Hill[110] found 2.6% of college athletes met the criteria for all 3 components. Torstveit and Sundgot-Borgen[111] found 4.3% of elite Europeans had evidence of all 3 components. Unfortunately, each study used different criteria for each component making comparisons between studies difficult.

Screening, Diagnosis, and Treatment

These data show that there is a high prevalence of the triad characteristics in a variety of ages and sports. Therefore, awareness, screening, treatment, and prevention are crucial, especially because the triad is a silent process and is easy to miss unless the practitioner has a high index of suspicion. The ACSM Position Stand recommends that screening for the triad be done at preparticipation examinations and at annual health examinations.[87] The ACSM also recommends that athletes with 1 component of the female athlete triad be assessed for the other components.[87] Screening may include history (information on energy intake, dietary practices, weight fluctuations, eating behaviors, and energy expenditure), physical examination (height, weight, body mass index [BMI, calculated as weight in kilograms divided by the square of height in meters], percent body fat, and vital signs), and laboratory screening (electrolytes, chemistry profile, complete blood count with differential, erythrocyte sedimentation rate, thyroid function tests, urinalysis, pregnancy test, follicle-stimulating hormone, luteinizing hormone, prolactin, free testosterone, dehydroepiandrosterone sulfate, and serum estradiol).[87] A BMD assessment by dual-energy absorptiometry should be considered after multiple stress fractures and/or 6 months of menstrual dysfunction or disordered eating with a machine that has a pediatric database.[87] Initial treatment of the female athlete triad is focused on increasing energy availability by increasing energy intake or by decreasing energy expenditure.[87] Oral contraceptive pills are controversial in the treatment of menstrual dysfunction. Some studies show a reduction in BMD, whereas others show maintenance of BMD. It is thought that taking oral contraceptives and having withdrawal bleeding may give runners a false sense that they are in a positive energy balance and their BMD is not at risk. Runners with low energy availability should be referred for nutritional assessment and dietary counseling by a registered dietitian with experience in treating female athletes.[87] Some athletes who have difficulty increasing calories or decreasing exercise may need to be referred for counseling or require serotonin reuptake inhibitors. The best treatment of the female athlete triad is prevention. This is optimally obtained from early education and increasing awareness of this disorder among our female athletes, parents, coaches, and health care providers. Preferably, this should start in middle school.

ENDOTHELIAL DYSFUNCTION/FOLIC ACID

The interrelationship between disordered eating, amenorrhea, and osteoporosis has been well established; however, there is increasing evidence of a fourth component, endovascular disease, in these athletes.

Cardiovascular Dysfunction

In the United States, the number 1 cause of death in women is cardiovascular disease; 1 in 4 will die of a cardiac event.[112] Cardiovascular disease increases significantly after menopause[112] when ovarian failure leads to decreased circulating estrogens. It is well known that in postmenopausal women, hypoestrogenism has harmful effects on endothelial function and cardiovascular health.[113–120] Hypoestrogenism is also believed to play a role in endothelial dysfunction in young amenorrheic runners.[121,122] Endogenous estrogens are known to be cardioprotective in reducing low-density lipoproteins, reducing total cholesterol, and increasing high-density lipoprotein levels.[123] In addition to an improved lipid profile, estrogen may have protective effects.[124] Vascular function is regulated partially by estrogen as vascular endothelial cells and smooth muscle cells have estrogen receptors. Estrogen has fast vasodilatory effects and slower longer-term effects that inhibit the vascular injury response helping to prevent atherosclerosis. These estrogen receptors are found on the vascular endothelium of coronary and peripheral vessels and estrogen can stimulate the production of nitric oxide in 2 ways. First, estrogen increases the production of endothelial-derived nitric oxide, which leads to vasodilation.[125–127] Second, estrogen stimulates genomic pathways, which involves changes in gene and protein expression, modulating the response to injury and atherosclerosis.[126] Nitric oxide is not only a potent vasodilator but also prevents platelet aggregation, leukocyte adhesion, and vascular smooth muscle proliferation and migration, each a key component of the atherosclerotic process.[128,129] Menopause, presumably secondary to low estrogen levels, is associated with reduced endothelium-dependent dilation,[130] which is not unlike the low estrogen levels in runners with athletic-associated menstrual dysfunction.

Endothelial Dysfunction

In cardiovascular disease, impaired endothelial function is likely the sentinel atherogenic event[131–133] and the earliest sign of cardiovascular disease.[131] Moreover, long-term atherosclerotic disease progression and cardiovascular event rates are predicted by vascular endothelial dysfunction.[134] Endothelial dysfunction can be seen as early as 3 months after menopause[113] and as early as 7 days after ovariectomy in premenopausal women.[135] Brachial artery endothelial dysfunction is strongly predictive of coronary artery endothelial dysfunction, making this a valid marker for cardiovascular disease risk.[136] Cardiovascular risk can be assessed by measuring flow-mediated dilation (FMD), which is an indirect measure of endothelial cell function. Using FMD, researchers have shown that premenopausal female runners with athletic-associated amenorrhea have reduced endothelial-dependent FMD of the brachial artery compared with eumenorrheic runners.[121,122,137] These studies found that the endothelial dysfunction of amenorrheic runners (aged 21.9 ± 1.2 years, mean $\pm$ SE) was similar to that of postmenopausal women (aged 60.0 ± 2.0 years) with known cardiovascular disease.[138] A study by Hoch and colleagues[121] found that eumenorrheic runners may also have reduced brachial artery dilation even though they have no apparent risk factors for cardiovascular disease. Most likely a critical level of estrogen exists that affects endothelial function independent of the presence or absence of menstrual bleeding. Based on these studies, runners with menstrual irregularities who have reduced endothelium-dependent dilation of the brachial artery may be predisposed to accelerated cardiovascular risk.

Reversibility of Endothelial Dysfunction

It is now known that athletic-associated amenorrhea is associated with endothelial dysfunction; however, is this dysfunction reversible? There are studies that support the hypothesis that estrogen exerts a cardioprotective effect via its interaction with the vascular endothelium in postmenopausal women.[113] More recently, studies have shown that oral contraceptive administration (30 μg ethinyl estradiol and 150 μg levonorgestrel) significantly improved brachial artery FMD in premenopausal amenorrheic runners.[122] However, the Women's Health Initiative (WHI) study found that postmenopausal women who were using hormone replacement therapy that included both estrogen and progestin had an increased risk of breast cancer, heart disease, stroke, and blood clots.[139,140] Many runners are not postmenopausal, however with the knowledge that was gained from the WHI, an alternative treatment approach to reduced brachial artery FMD in amenorrheic runners is warranted. One such therapy to consider is folic acid.

Folic Acid

Folic acid improves cardiovascular parameters including endothelial function, arterial stiffness, blood pressure, and thrombotic activity.[141–149] Several studies found that folic acid supplementation improved endothelial function in numerous disease states, including hypercholesterolemia,[150,151] hypertension,[143] diabetes,[152] coronary artery disease,[153,154] and cardiovascular disease.[155] In addition, folic acid has shown benefit in Alzheimer disease and the prevention of colon cancer and neural tube defects.[155] These studies suggest that higher folic acid intake may have vasculoprotective effects in certain patient populations.

There are 2 types of endothelial vasodilation; endothelial-dependent vasodilatation and endothelium-independent vasodilation. Folic acid improves endothelial-dependent vasodilatation in men with hypertension, coronary artery disease, congestive heart failure, and peripheral vascular disease.[151,156–160] Moreover, some studies indicate that there is no significant difference in endothelium-independent vasodilation between amenorrheic, oligomenorrheic, and eumenorrheic women.[121]

There are multiple mechanisms to explain how folic acid supplementation improves endothelial-dependent vasodilatation. First, folic acid may have a direct antioxidant effect in the vasculature, increasing NO bioavailability and improving FMD.[161] Second, it is believed that folates participate in the endogenous regeneration of tetrahydrobiopterin,[162] which is an essential cofactor for endothelial nitric oxide synthase (eNOS) to produce nitric oxide (NO). With increased levels of tetrahydrobiopterin, there will likely be increased NO production. Third, the homocysteine-lowering effect of folic acid can contribute to improvements in endothelial function[163,164]; however, some studies have shown that folic acid improves endothelial function without producing significant changes in homocysteine concentration.[142,145,150]

Most recently, studies have shown that runners treated with folic acid had improved endothelial-dependent vasodilatation. One study by Hoch and colleagues[165] found that folic acid supplementation (10 mg/d) for 4 to 6 weeks significantly improved endothelial-dependent FMD in eumenorrheic women runners with normal folic acid levels compared with a placebo control group. Another study by Hoch and colleagues[166] found that 4 weeks of folic acid supplementation improved brachial artery FMD in amenorrheic runners.

Although it is known that folic acid is beneficial for cardiovascular parameters, the optimal dose has not been identified. Folic acid is a water-soluble vitamin that is regularly eliminated in the urine. For women aged 19 to 50 years, the recommended daily allowance for folate is 400 μg/d and the tolerable upper intake level (UL) is 1 g/d. The UL refers to the amount of synthetic folate (folic acid) being consumed per day from fortified foods and/or supplements. There are no health risks and no UL for natural sources of folate found in food and the risk of toxicity from folic acid intake from supplements and/or fortified foods is low.[167] Increased folic acid is recommended in some populations. Four milligrams of folate per day is recommended for women who have risk factors for neural tube defects. Multiple studies have shown that 10 mg of folic acid daily is safe and improves FMD.[160,165,166,168–171] At 10 mg of folic acid per day, there have been no reported side effects[160,168–171] and the US Food and Drug Administration MedWatch system does not list any adverse effects of folic acid at this dose in runners.[171] Side effects such as upset stomach, sleep disturbances, and skin problems have been noted at higher doses (>15 mg/d).

Even though there are benefits of folic acid supplementation, high levels of folic acid can pose a variety of health risks to some individuals. For instance, high doses of folic acid can bring about seizures in patients who also taking anticonvulsant medications.[172] According to the National Institutes of Health (NIH), patients with a vitamin B_{12} deficiency need to use caution with folic acid as it may hide the deficiency and silently worsen the disease.[173] According to a recent study in patients with a known history of colorectal adenomas, folic acid supplementation may increase the risk of recurrent colorectal adenoma.[174]

In many runners, the benefits of folic acid supplementation may outweigh the risks, especially in those runners opposed to estrogen supplementation. Clinicians can potentially recommend folic acid on a daily basis to runners with menstrual dysfunction if brachial artery FMD is found to be low; however, the optimal dose is yet to be determined.

SUMMARY

Female athletes, especially runners, have come a long way in the last several decades. There are millions of female runners today, and it is important to be aware of the significant anatomic, physiologic, and psychological issues facing the female runner. Female runners have special issues in relation to pregnancy and aging. The female athlete triad is a critical, complex physiologic, and often psychological, condition that affects young runners. Cardiovascular dysfunction not uncommonly accompanies the female athlete triad, making a compelling argument for the female athlete tetrad consisting of disordered eating, amenorrhea, osteoporosis, and cardiovascular dysfunction. Oral folic acid treatment may be a safe and inexpensive method to improve endothelial dysfunction in female runners.

REFERENCES

1. US Department of Labor. Title IX, Education amendments of 1972. Available at: http://www.dol.gov/oasam/regs/statutes/titleIX.htm. Accessed June 5, 2009.
2. NFSHSA. 2005-06 High School Athletics Participation Survey: based on competition at the high school level in 2005-06 school year. National Federation of State High Schools. Kansas City (MO): The National Federation of States High Schools Association Handbook; 2006.
3. Gender equity in intercollegiate athletics: a practical guide for colleges and universities - 2008. Indianapolis (IN): National Collegiate Athletic Association; 2008. Available at: http://www.ncaapublications.com/p-4023-gender-equity-in-intercollegiate-athletics-2008.aspx. Accessed June 15, 2009.
4. Lopiano D. Gender equity in sports. In: Agostini R, editor. Medical and orthopedic issues of active and athletic women. Philadelphia: Hanley & Belfus; 1994. p. 13–22.
5. Burton NM. The stronger women get, the more men love football: sexism and the American culture of sports. Arlington (VA): Dare Press; 2005.
6. Thomas K. A city team's struggle shows disparity in girls' sports. 2009. Available at: http://www.nytimes.com/2009/06/14/sports/14girls.html?_r=3&th&emc=th. 2009. Accessed June 15, 2009.
7. Beijing Organizing Committee for the Games of the XXIX Olympiad. Official website of the Beijing 2008 Olympic Games: record women's participation. Available at: http://en.beijing2008.cn/news/official/ioc/n214559789.shtml. 2008. Accessed June 19, 2009.
8. United States Olympic Committee. 2008 United States Olympic Team entered into XXVIV Olympic Games in Beijing, China. 2008. Available at: http://teamusa.org/news/article/2744. Accessed June 19, 2009.
9. NBC Universal. Team USA: track and field - women. Available at: http://www.nbcolympics.com/teamusa/meettheteam/newsid=114076.html. Accessed June 19, 2009.
10. NBC Universal. Team USA: track and field - men. Available at: http://www.nbcolympics.com/teamusa/meettheteam/newsid=114075.html#track+field+men. Accessed June 19, 2009.
11. United States Olympic Committee. Competition information: metal standings - athletics. 2008. Available at: http://results.beijing2008.cn/WRM/ENG/INF/AT/C95/AT0000000.shtml. Accessed June 19, 2009.
12. MarketResearch.com. The U.S. market for women's athletic apparel. 2001. Available at: http://www.marketresearch.com/product/display.asp?productid=186555&xs=r. Accessed June 12, 2009.
13. Van Riper T, Badenhausen K. Top earning female athletes. 2008. Available at: http://www.forbes.com/2008/07/22/women-athletes-endorsements-biz-sports-cx_tvr_kb_0722athletes.html. Accessed June 30, 3009.
14. Taimela S, Kujala UM, Osterman K. Intrinsic risk factors and athletic injuries. Sports Med 1990;9(4):205–15.
15. Greydanus DE, Patel DR. The female athlete. Before and beyond puberty. Pediatr Clin North Am 2002;49(3):553–80.
16. Hewett TE, Myer GD, Ford KR. Decrease in neuromuscular control about the knee with maturation in female athletes. J Bone Joint Surg Am 2004;86(8):1601–8.

17. Bailey DA, Martin AD, McKay HA, et al. Calcium accretion in girls and boys during puberty: a longitudinal analysis. J Bone Miner Res 2000;15(11):2245–50.

18. Natural Hormones. About testosterone. Available at: http://www.natural-hormones.net/testosterone-about.htm. Accessed August 7, 2009.

19. Cureton KJ, Collins MA, Hill DW, et al. Muscle hypertrophy in men and women. Med Sci Sports Exerc 1988;20(4):338–44.

20. Ebben W, Jensen R. Strength training in women: debunking myths that block opportunity. Phys Sportsmed 1998;26:86–97.

21. Huston LJ, Wojtys EM. Neuromuscular performance characteristics in elite female athletes. Am J Sports Med 1996;24(4):427–36.

22. Yurko-Griffin L, Harris S. Female athletes. In: Sullivan J, Anderson S, editors. Care of the young athlete. Rosemont (IL): American Academy of Orthopaedic Surgeons; 1999. p. 137–48.

23. Malina RM. Body composition in athletes: assessment and estimated fatness. Clin Sports Med 2007;26(1):37–68.

24. Noakes TD. The lore of running. Champaign (IL): Leisure Press; 1991.

25. Wells C. Women, sport and performance: a physiological perspective. Champaign (IL): Human Kinetics; 1991. p. 3–34.

26. Torstveit MK, Sundgot-Borgen J. Low bone mineral density is two to three times more prevalent in non-athletic premenopausal women than in elite athletes: a comprehensive controlled study. Br J Sports Med 2005;39(5):282–7.

27. Hoch AZ, Pajewski NM, Moraski L, et al. Prevalence of the female athlete triad in high school athletes and sedentary students. Clin J Sport Med 2009;19(5): 421–8.

28. Kannus P, Haapasalo H, Sankelo M, et al. Effect of starting age of physical activity on bone mass in the dominant arm of tennis and squash players. Ann Intern Med 1995;123(1):27–31.

29. Duncan CS, Blimkie CJ, Cowell CT, et al. Bone mineral density in adolescent female athletes: relationship to exercise type and muscle strength. Med Sci Sports Exerc 2002;34(2):286–94.

30. Lloyd T, Chinchilli VM, Eggli DF, et al. Body composition development of adolescent white females: the Penn State Young Women's Health Study. Arch Pediatr Adolesc Med 1998;152(10):998–1002.

31. Tanner J. Growth at adolescence. Oxford: Blackwell Publishers Ltd; 1962.

32. Hale R. Factors important to women engaged in regular physical activity. In: Strauss R, editor. Sports medicine and physiology. Philadelphia: WB Saunders; 1984. p. 250–69.

33. Marshall J. Myths about women's sports. In: Marshall J, editor. The sports doctor's fitness book for women. New York: Delacorte; 1981. p. 6–13.

34. Astrand P, Rodahl K. Textbook of work physiology: physiological bases of exercise. New York: McGraw-Hill; 1977.

35. DeVries H. Physiology of exercise for physical education and athletics. Dubuque (IA): WC Brown Co; 1980.

36. Guenette JA, Witt JD, McKenzie DC, et al. Respiratory mechanics during exercise in endurance-trained men and women. J Physiol 2007;581(Pt 3):1309–22.

37. Cureton KJ, Sparling PB. Distance running performance and metabolic responses to running in men and women with excess weight experimentally equated. Med Sci Sports Exerc 1980;12(4):288–94.

38. Cureton K, Bishop P, Hutchinson P, et al. Sex difference in maximal oxygen uptake. Effect of equating haemoglobin concentration. Eur J Appl Physiol Occup Physiol 1986;54(6):656–60.

39. Prather H, Hunt D. Issues unique to the female runner. Phys Med Rehabil Clin N Am 2005;16(3):691–709.

40. Shultz SJ, Perrin DH. Using surface electromyography to assess sex differences in neuromuscular response characteristics. J Athl Train 1999;34(2):165–76.

41. Rozzi SL, Lephart SM, Gear WS, et al. Knee joint laxity and neuromuscular characteristics of male and female soccer and basketball players. Am J Sports Med 1999;27(3):312–9.

42. Dugan SA. Sports-related knee injuries in female athletes: what gives? Am J Phys Med Rehabil 2005;84(2):122–30.

43. Arnheim D. Modern principles of athletic training. St. Louis (MO): Mosby; 1989.

44. Thomas C. Factors important to women participants in vigorous athletics. In: Strauss R, editor. Sports medicine and physiology. Philadelphia: WB Saunders; 1979. p. 304–19.

45. Atwater A. Biomechanics and the female athlete. In: Puhl J, Brown C, Voy R, editors. Sports science perspectives for women. Champaign (IL): Human Kinetics; 1988. p. 1–12.

46. Klafs C, Lyon M. The female athlete: a coach's guide to conditioning and training. St. Louis (MO): CV Mosby Co; 1978. p. 15–46.

47. Ireland ML, Willson JD, Ballantyne BT, et al. Hip strength in females with and without patellofemoral pain. J Orthop Sports Phys Ther 2003;33(11):671–6.

48. Ferber R, Hreljac A, Kendall S. Suspected mechanism in the cause of overuse running injuries: a clinical review. Sports Health: A Multidisciplinary Approach 2009;1(3):242–6. Available at: http://sph.sagepub.com/. Accessed March 5, 2010.

49. Horton M, Hall T. Quadriceps femoris muscle angle: normal values and relationships with gender and selected skeletal measures. Phys Ther 1989;69:897–901.

50. Fredericson M, Cookingham CL, Chaudhari AM, et al. Hip abductor weakness in distance runners with iliotibial band syndrome. Clin J Sport Med 2000;10(3):169–75.

51. Earl J, Hoch AZ, Labisch T, et al. Patient outcomes, strength and lower extremity biomechanics following a proximal rehabilitation program in women with patellofemoral pain syndrome. J Athl Train 2008;43(3):S51.

52. Landry SC, McKean KA, Hubley-Kozey CL, et al. Neuromuscular and lower limb biomechanical differences exist between male and female elite adolescent soccer players during an unanticipated run and crosscut maneuver. Am J Sports Med 2007;35(11):1901–11.

53. Davidson D, Welborn T, Azure D, et al. Male and female body shape preferences of young children in the United States, Main Land China and Turkey. Child Study 2002;32(3):131–3.

54. McCabe MP, Ricciardelli LA. A prospective study of pressures from parents, peers, and the media on extreme weight change behaviors among adolescent boys and girls. Behav Res Ther 2005;43(5):653–68.

55. Phares V, Steinberg A, Thompson K. Gender differences in peer and parental influences: body image disturbances, self-worth and psychological functioning in preadolescent children. J Youth Adolesc 2004;33(5):421–9.

56. Schur EA, Sanders M, Steiner H. Body dissatisfaction and dieting in young children. Int J Eat Disord 2000;27(1):74–82.

57. Sundgot-Borgen J. Risk and trigger factors for the development of eating disorders in female elite athletes. Med Sci Sports Exerc 1994;26(4):414–9.

58. Zhang J, Savitz DA. Exercise during pregnancy among US women. Ann Epidemiol 1996;6(1):53–9.

59. Clapp JF III. Long-term outcome after exercising throughout pregnancy: fitness and cardiovascular risk. Am J Obstet Gynecol 2008;199(5):489.

60. Symons Downs D, Hausenblas HA. Women's exercise beliefs and behaviors during their pregnancy and postpartum. J Midwifery Womens Health 2004; 49(2):138–44.

61. Hale RW, Milne L. The elite athlete and exercise in pregnancy. Semin Perinatol 1996;20(4):277–84.

62. Lof M, Forsum E. Activity pattern and energy expenditure due to physical activity before and during pregnancy in healthy Swedish women. Br J Nutr 2006;95(2): 296–302.

63. ACOG Committee Obstetric Practice. ACOG Committee opinion. Number 267, January 2002: exercise during pregnancy and the postpartum period. Obstet Gynecol 2002;99(1):171–3.

64. Holschen JC. The female athlete. South Med J 2004;97(9):852–8.

65. Clapp JF III, Kim H, Burciu B, et al. Continuing regular exercise during pregnancy: effect of exercise volume on fetoplacental growth. Am J Obstet Gynecol 2002;186(1):142–7.

66. Bergmann A, Zygmunt M, Clapp JF III. Running throughout pregnancy: effect on placental villous vascular volume and cell proliferation. Placenta 2004;25(8–9): 694–8.

67. Kardel KR, Kase T. Training in pregnant women: effects on fetal development and birth. Am J Obstet Gynecol 1998;178(2):280–6.

68. Clapp JF III, Simonian S, Lopez B, et al. The one-year morphometric and neurodevelopmental outcome of the offspring of women who continued to exercise regularly throughout pregnancy. Am J Obstet Gynecol 1998;178(3): 594–9.

69. Beilock SL, Feltz DL, Pivarnik JM. Training patterns of athletes during pregnancy and postpartum. Res Q Exerc Sport 2001;72(1):39–46.

70. Clapp JF III, Capeless E. The VO2max of recreational athletes before and after pregnancy. Med Sci Sports Exerc 1991;23(10):1128–33.

71. Artal R, O'Toole M. Guidelines of the American College of Obstetricians and Gynecologists for exercise during pregnancy and the postpartum period. Br J Sports Med 2003;37(1):6–12.

72. Milsom I, Abrams P, Cardozo L, et al. How widespread are the symptoms of an overactive bladder and how are they managed? A population-based prevalence study. BJU Int 2001;87(9):760–6.

73. Hannestad YS, Rortveit G, Sandvik H, et al. A community-based epidemiological survey of female urinary incontinence: the Norwegian EPINCONT study. Epidemiology of Incontinence in the County of Nord-Trondelag. J Clin Epidemiol 2000;53(11):1150–7.

74. Bo K, Borgen JS. Prevalence of stress and urge urinary incontinence in elite athletes and controls. Med Sci Sports Exerc 2001;33(11):1797–802.

75. Zhu L, Lang J, Wang H, et al. The prevalence of and potential risk factors for female urinary incontinence in Beijing, China. Menopause 2008;15(3):566–9.

76. Crepin G, Biserte J, Cosson M, et al. The female urogenital system and high level sports. Bull Acad Natl Med 2006;190(7):1479–91.

77. Warren MP, Shantha S. The female athlete. Baillieres Best Pract Res Clin Endocrinol Metab 2000;14(1):37–53.

78. Carls C. The prevalence of stress urinary incontinence in high school and college-age female athletes in the midwest: implications for education and prevention. Urol Nurs 2007;27(1):21–4, 39.

79. Nygaard IE, Thompson FL, Svengalis SL, et al. Urinary incontinence in elite nulliparous athletes. Obstet Gynecol 1994;84(2):183–7.

80. Nygaard IE. Does prolonged high-impact activity contribute to later urinary incontinence? A retrospective cohort study of female Olympians. Obstet Gynecol 1997;90(5):718–22.

81. Mayo Foundation. Urinary incontinence. 2009. Available at: http://www.mayoclinic.com/health/urinary-incontinence/DS00404/DSECTION=treatments-and-drugs. Accessed July 27, 2009.

82. Helmick CG, Felson DT, Lawrence RC, et al. Estimates of the prevalence of arthritis and other rheumatic conditions in the United States. Part I. Arthritis Rheum 2008;58(1):15–25.

83. Lawrence RC, Helmick CG, Arnett FC, et al. Estimates of the prevalence of arthritis and selected musculoskeletal disorders in the United States. Arthritis Rheum 1998;41(5):778–99.

84. Arthritis Foundation. News from the Arthritis Foundation: osteoarthritis fact sheet. Available at: http://www.arthritis.org/media/newsroom/media-kits/Osteoarthritis_fact_sheet.pdf. Accessed July 27, 2009.

85. Felson DT, Niu J, Clancy M, et al. Effect of recreational physical activities on the development of knee osteoarthritis in older adults of different weights: the Framingham Study. Arthritis Rheum 2007;57(1):6–12.

86. Felson DT, Zhang Y, Anthony JM, et al. Weight loss reduces the risk for symptomatic knee osteoarthritis in women. The Framingham Study. Ann Intern Med 1992;116(7):535–9.

87. Nattiv A, Loucks AB, Manore MM, et al. American College of Sports Medicine position stand. The female athlete triad. Med Sci Sports Exerc 2007;39(10):1867–82.

88. Sundgot-Borgen J. Nutrient intake of female elite athletes suffering from eating disorders. Int J Sport Nutr 1993;3(4):431–42.

89. Wade GN, Schneider JE, Li HY. Control of fertility by metabolic cues. Am J Physiol 1996;270(1 Pt 1):E1–19.

90. Kaiserauer S, Snyder AC, Sleeper M, et al. Nutritional, physiological, and menstrual status of distance runners. Med Sci Sports Exerc 1989;21(2):120–5.

91. Marcus R, Cann C, Madvig P, et al. Menstrual function and bone mass in elite women distance runners. Endocrine and metabolic features. Ann Intern Med 1985;102(2):158–63.

92. Practice Committee of the American Society for Reproductive Medicine. Current evaluation of amenorrhea. Fertil Steril 2004;82(1):266–72.

93. De Souza MJ, Williams NI. Physiological aspects and clinical sequelae of energy deficiency and hypoestrogenism in exercising women. Hum Reprod Update 2004;10(5):433–48.

94. Loucks AB, Thuma JR. Luteinizing hormone pulsatility is disrupted at a threshold of energy availability in regularly menstruating women. J Clin Endocrinol Metab 2003;88(1):297–311.

95. Golden NH, Carlson JL. The pathophysiology of amenorrhea in the adolescent. Ann N Y Acad Sci 2008;113:5163–78.

96. Meczekalski B, Podfigurna-Stopa A, Warenik-Szymankiewicz A, et al. Functional hypothalamic amenorrhea: current view on neuroendocrine aberrations. Gynecol Endocrinol 2008;24(1):4–11.

97. Rigotti NA, Nussbaum SR, Herzog DB, et al. Osteoporosis in women with anorexia nervosa. N Engl J Med 1984;311(25):1601–6.

98. Drinkwater BL, Bruemner B, Chesnut CH. Menstrual history as a determinant of current bone density in young athletes. JAMA 1990;263(4):545–8.

99. Robinson TL, Snow-Harter C, Taaffe DR, et al. Gymnasts exhibit higher bone mass than runners despite similar prevalence of amenorrhea and oligomenorrhea. J Bone Miner Res 1995;10(1):26–35.
100. Risser WL, Lee EJ, LeBlanc A, et al. Bone density in eumenorrheic female college athletes. Med Sci Sports Exerc 1990;22(5):570–4.
101. Weaver CM. The role of nutrition on optimizing peak bone mass. Asia Pac J Clin Nutr 2008;17(Suppl):1135–7.
102. Ihle R, Loucks AB. Dose-response relationships between energy availability and bone turnover in young exercising women. J Bone Miner Res 2004;19(8): 1231–40.
103. Khan K, McKay H, Kannus P, et al. Physical activity and bone health. Champaign (IL): Human Kinetics; 2001.
104. Hoch AZ, Stavrakos JE, Schimke JE. Prevalence of female athlete triad characteristics in club triathlon team. Arch Phys Med Rehabil 2007;88(5):681–2.
105. Thompson SH. Characteristics of the female athlete triad in collegiate cross-country runners. J Am Coll Health 2007;56(2):129–36.
106. Torstveit MK, Rosenvinge JH, Sundgot-Borgen J. Prevalence of eating disorders and the predictive power of risk models in female elite athletes: a controlled study. Scand J Med Sci Sports 2008;18(1):108–18.
107. Dusek T. Influence of high intensity training on menstrual cycle disorders in athletes. Croat Med J 2001;42(1):79–82.
108. Nichols JF, Rauh MJ, Lawson MJ, et al. Prevalence of the female athlete triad syndrome among high school athletes. Arch Pediatr Adolesc Med 2006; 160(2):137–42.
109. Wiksten-Almstromer M, Hirschberg AL, Hagenfeldt K. Reduced bone mineral density in adult women diagnosed with menstrual disorders during adolescence. Acta Obstet Gynecol Scand 2009;88(5):543–9.
110. Beals KA, Hill AK. The prevalence of disordered eating, menstrual dysfunction, and low bone mineral density among US collegiate athletes. Int J Sport Nutr Exerc Metab 2006;16(1):1–23.
111. Torstveit MK, Sundgot-Borgen J. The female athlete triad exists in both elite athletes and controls. Med Sci Sports Exerc 2005;37(9):1449–59.
112. Barrett-Connor E, Bush TL. Estrogen and coronary heart disease in women. JAMA 1991;265(14):1861–7.
113. Lieberman EH, Gerhard MD, Uehata A, et al. Estrogen improves endothelium-dependent, flow-mediated vasodilation in postmenopausal women. Ann Intern Med 1994;121:936–41.
114. Mijatovic V, Kenemans P, Jakobs C, et al. A randomized controlled study of the effects of 17beta-estradiol-dydrogesterone on plasma homocysteine in postmenopausal women. Obstet Gynecol 1998;91(3):432–6.
115. Moreau KL, Donato AJ, Tanaka H, et al. Basal leg blood flow in healthy women is related to age and hormone replacement therapy status. J Physiol 2003; 547(Pt 1):309–16.
116. Ridker PM, Hennekens CH, Buring JE, et al. C-reactive protein and other markers of inflammation in the prediction of cardiovascular disease in women. N Engl J Med 2000;342(12):836–43.
117. Rosenson RS, Tangney CC, Mosca LJ. Hormone replacement therapy improves cardiovascular risk by lowering plasma viscosity in postmenopausal women. Arterioscler Thromb Vasc Biol 1998;18(12):1902–5.
118. Stevenson JC, Crook D, Godsland IF. Influence of age and menopause on serum lipids and lipoproteins in healthy women. Atherosclerosis 1993;98(1):83–90.

119. Yen CH, Hsieh CC, Chou SY, et al. 17Beta-estradiol inhibits oxidized low density lipoprotein-induced generation of reactive oxygen species in endothelial cells. Life Sci 2001;70(4):403–13.

120. Yildirir A, Aybar F, Tokgozoglu L, et al. Effects of hormone replacement therapy on plasma homocysteine and C-reactive protein levels. Gynecol Obstet Invest 2002;53(1):54–8.

121. Hoch AZ, Dempsey RL, Carrera GF, et al. Is there an association between athletic amenorrhea and endothelial cell dysfunction? Med Sci Sports Exerc 2003;35(3):377–83.

122. Rickenlund A, Eriksson MJ, Schenck-Gustafsson K, et al. Oral contraceptives improve endothelial function in amenorrheic athletes. J Clin Endocrinol Metab 2005;90(6):3162–7.

123. Walsh BW, Schiff I, Rosner B, et al. Effects of postmenopausal estrogen replacement on the concentrations and metabolism of plasma lipoproteins. N Engl J Med 1991;325(17):1196–204.

124. Bush TL, Barrett-Connor E, Cowan LD, et al. Cardiovascular mortality and non-contraceptive use of estrogen in women: results from the Lipid Research Clinics Program Follow-up Study. Circulation 1987;75(6):1102–9.

125. Cid MC, Schnaper HW, Kleinman HK. Estrogens and the vascular endothelium. Ann N Y Acad Sci 2002;966:143–57.

126. Mendelsohn ME. Protective effects of estrogen on the cardiovascular system. Am J Cardiol 2002;89(12A):12E–7E.

127. Schnaper HW, McGuire J, Runyan C, et al. Sex steroids and the endothelium. Curr Med Chem 2000;7(5):519–31.

128. Moncada S, Higgs A. The L-arginine-nitric oxide pathway. N Engl J Med 1993; 329:2002–12.

129. Dusting GJ, Fennessy P, Yin ZL, et al. Nitric oxide in atherosclerosis: vascular protector or villain? Clin Exp Pharmacol Physiol Suppl 1998;25:S34–41.

130. Perregaux D, Chaudhuri A, Mohanty P, et al. Effect of gender differences and estrogen replacement therapy on vascular reactivity. Metabolism 1999;48(2): 227–32.

131. Celermajer DS. Endothelial dysfunction: does it matter? Is it reversible? J Am Coll Cardiol 1997;30:325–33.

132. Ganz P, Vita JA. Testing endothelial vasomotor function: nitric oxide, a multipotent molecule. Circulation 2003;108(17):2049–53.

133. Ross R. Atherosclerosis–an inflammatory disease. N Engl J Med 1999;340(2): 115–26.

134. Schachinger V, Britten MB, Zeiher AM. Prognostic impact of coronary vasodilator dysfunction on adverse long- term outcome of coronary heart disease. Circulation 2000;101(16):1899–906.

135. Ohmichi M, Kanda Y, Hisamoto K, et al. Rapid changes of flow-mediated dilatation after surgical menopause. Maturitas 2003;44(2):125–31.

136. Anderson TJ, Uehata A, Gerhard MD, et al. Close relation of endothelial function in the human coronary and peripheral circulations. J Am Coll Cardiol 1995;26: 1235–41.

137. Rickenlund A, Eriksson MJ, Schenck-Gustafsson K, et al. Amenorrhea in female athletes is associated with endothelial dysfunction and unfavorable lipid profile. J Clin Endocrinol Metab 2005;90(3):1354–9.

138. Celermajer DS, Sorensen KE, Gooch VM, et al. Non-invasive detection of endothelial dysfunction in children and adults at risk of atherosclerosis. Lancet 1992; 340(8828):1111–5.

139. Rossouw JE, Anderson GL, Prentice RL, et al. Risks and benefits of estrogen plus progestin in healthy postmenopausal women: principal results From the Women's Health Initiative randomized controlled trial. JAMA 2002;288(3):321–33.
140. Heiss G, Wallace R, Anderson GL, et al. Health risks and benefits 3 years after stopping randomized treatment with estrogen and progestin. JAMA 2008; 299(9):1036–45.
141. Schutte AE, Huisman HW, Oosthuizen W, et al. Cardiovascular effects of oral supplementation of vitamin C, E and folic acid in young healthy males. Int J Vitam Nutr Res 2004;74(4):285–93.
142. Mangoni AA, Sherwood RA, Swift CG, et al. Folic acid enhances endothelial function and reduces blood pressure in smokers: a randomized controlled trial. J Intern Med 2002;252(6):497–503.
143. van Dijk RA, Rauwerda JA, Steyn M, et al. Long-term homocysteine-lowering treatment with folic acid plus pyridoxine is associated with decreased blood pressure but not with improved brachial artery endothelium-dependent vasodilation or carotid artery stiffness: a 2-year, randomized, placebo-controlled trial. Arterioscler Thromb Vasc Biol 2001;21(12):2072–9.
144. Chambers JC, Ueland PM, Obeid OA, et al. Improved vascular endothelial function after oral B vitamins: an effect mediated through reduced concentrations of free plasma homocysteine. Circulation 2000;102(20):2479–83.
145. Mangoni AA, Sherwood RA, Asonganyi B, et al. Short-term oral folic acid supplementation enhances endothelial function in patients with type 2 diabetes. Am J Hypertens 2005;18(2 Pt 1):220–6.
146. Mangoni AA, Ouldred E, Swif CG, et al. Vascular and blood pressure effects of folic acid in older patients with cardiovascular disease. J Am Geriatr Soc 2001; 49(7):1003–4.
147. Deol PS, Barnes TA, Dampier K, et al. The effects of folic acid supplements on coagulation status in pregnancy. Br J Haematol 2004;127(2):204–8.
148. Undas A, Domagala TB, Jankowski M, et al. Treatment of hyperhomocysteinemia with folic acid and vitamins B12 and B6 attenuates thrombin generation. Thromb Res 1999;95(6):281–8.
149. Mangoni AA, Arya R, Ford E, et al. Effects of folic acid supplementation on inflammatory and thrombogenic markers in chronic smokers. A randomised controlled trial. Thromb Res 2003;110(1):13–7.
150. Verhaar MC, Wever RM, Kastelein JJ, et al. 5-Methyltetrahydrofolate, the active form of folic acid, restores endothelial function in familial hypercholesterolemia. Circulation 1998;97(3):237–41.
151. Verhaar MC, Wever RM, Kastelein JJ, et al. Effects of oral folic acid supplementation on endothelial function in familial hypercholesterolemia: a randomized placebo-controlled trial. Circulation 1999;100:335–8.
152. van Etten RW, de Koning EJ, Verhaar MC, et al. Impaired NO-dependent vasodilation in patients with Type II (non-insulin-dependent) diabetes mellitus is restored by acute administration of folate. Diabetologia 2002;45(7):1004–10.
153. Doshi SN, McDowell IF, Moat SJ, et al. Folate improves endothelial function in coronary artery disease: an effect mediated by reduction of intracellular superoxide? Arterioscler Thromb Vasc Biol 2001;21(7):1196–202.
154. Doshi SN, McDowell IF, Moat SJ, et al. Folic acid improves endothelial function in coronary artery disease via mechanisms largely independent of homocysteine lowering. Circulation 2002;105(1):22–6.
155. Birnbacher R, Messerschmidt AM, Pollak AP. Diagnosis and prevention of neural tube defects. Curr Opin Urol 2002;12(6):461–4.

156. Maxwell AJ, Anderson BE, Cooke JP. Nutritional therapy for peripheral arterial disease: a double-blind, placebo-controlled, randomized trial of HeartBar. Vasc Med 2000;5(1):11–9.

157. Boger RH, Bode-Boger SM, Thiele W, et al. Restoring vascular nitric oxide formation by L-arginine improves the symptoms of intermittent claudication in patients with peripheral arterial occlusive disease. J Am Coll Cardiol 1998; 32(5):1336–44.

158. Lekakis JP, Papathanassiou S, Papaioannou TG, et al. Oral L-arginine improves endothelial dysfunction in patients with essential hypertension. Int J Cardiol 2002;86(2–3):317–23.

159. Hambrecht R, Hilbrich L, Erbs S, et al. Correction of endothelial dysfunction in chronic heart failure: additional effects of exercise training and oral L-arginine supplementation. J Am Coll Cardiol 2000;35(3):706–13.

160. Wilmink HW, Stroes ES, Erkelens WD, et al. Influence of folic acid on postprandial endothelial dysfunction. Arterioscler Thromb Vasc Biol 2000;20(1):185–8.

161. Bonetti PO, Lerman LO, Lerman A. Endothelial dysfunction: a marker of atherosclerotic risk. Arterioscler Thromb Vasc Biol 2003;23(2):168–75.

162. Wever RM, van Dam T, van Rijn HJ, et al. Tetrahydrobiopterin regulates superoxide and nitric oxide generation by recombinant endothelial nitric oxide synthase. Biochem Biophys Res Commun 1997;237(2):340–4.

163. Pancharuniti N, Lewis CA, Sauberlich HE, et al. Plasma homocyst(e)ine, folate, and vitamin B-12 concentrations and risk for early-onset coronary artery disease. Am J Clin Nutr 1994;59(4):940–8.

164. van den BM, Boers GH, Franken DG, et al. Hyperhomocysteinaemia and endothelial dysfunction in young patients with peripheral arterial occlusive disease. Eur J Clin Invest 1995;25(3):176–81.

165. Hoch AZ, Pajewski NM, Hoffmann RG, et al. Possible relationship of folic acid supplementation and improved flow-mediated dilation in premenopausal, eumenorrheic athletic women. J Sports Sci Med 2009;81:23–9.

166. Hoch AZ, Lynch SL, Jurva JW, et al. Folic acid supplementation improves vascular function in amenorrheic runners. Clin J Sport Med 2010;20(3):205–10.

167. Hathcock JN. Vitamins and minerals: efficacy and safety. Am J Clin Nutr 1997; 66(2):427–37.

168. Moens AL, Claeys MJ, Wuyts FL, et al. Effect of folic acid on endothelial function following acute myocardial infarction. Am J Cardiol 2007;99(4):476–81.

169. Title LM, Ur E, Giddens K, et al. Folic acid improves endothelial dysfunction in type 2 diabetes–an effect independent of homocysteine-lowering. Vasc Med 2006;11(2):101–9.

170. Woo KS, Chook P, Lolin YI, et al. Folic acid improves arterial endothelial function in adults with hyperhomocystinemia. J Am Coll Cardiol 1999;34(7):2002–6.

171. US Food and Drug Administration. The FDA Safety Information and Adverse Event Reporting Program: medical product safety information. Available at: http://www.fda.gov/medwatch/SAFETY.htm. Accessed December 8, 2008.

172. Herbert V. Folic acid. In: Shils M, Olson J, Shike M, et al, editors. Modern nutrition in health and disease. Baltimore (MD): Williams & Wilkins; 1999. p. 433–66.

173. National Institutes of Health. Dietary supplement fact sheet: folate. 2007. Available at: http://ods.od.nih.gov/factsheets/folate.asp. Accessed June 12, 2009.

174. Cole BF, Baron JA, Sandler RS, et al. Folic acid for the prevention of colorectal adenomas: a randomized clinical trial. JAMA 2007;297(21):2351–9.

Pediatric Running Injuries

Craig K. Seto, MD*, Siobhan M. Statuta, MD, Ian L. Solari, MD

KEYWORDS

• Athlete • Overuse injury • Apophysis • Overtraining • Pediatric

The young athletic population continues to grow in the United States, with an estimated 30 to 35 million children aged 5 to 18 years participating in organized sports. Similarly, there has been an increase in the number of children participating in recreational and competitive running events nationwide.[1–4] Data from the National Federation of High Schools reported 429,000 young athletes participating in cross-country during 2008 to 2009, reflecting a steady increase from the 364,000 participants reported in 2003 to 2004.[5] With this increase in athletic participation there has also been a concomitant increase in the incidence of acute and overuse injuries in the young athletic population.[1] Most injuries in young runners are caused by overtraining, resulting in an overuse injury. These injuries are related to repetitive stress on the musculoskeletal system without sufficient recovery time, which overwhelms the normal reparative processes. In young runners, overuse injuries are often seen during sudden increases in the training regimen, which could include total mileage, intensity of running pace, or both. These increases commonly occur during sports camps and at the beginning of a new season.[1,3] Risk factors associated with overuse injuries in runners can be divided into intrinsic and extrinsic factors. Intrinsic factors include individual biomechanical factors such as lower extremity malalignment, leg length discrepancy, foot hyperpronation, muscle inflexibility or imbalance, and the female gender. Extrinsic factors include hard training surfaces, inappropriate or worn out running shoes, and training errors. It is important to address these risk factors when evaluating a young runner with an overuse injury.[1]

In the literature, there are few epidemiologic studies on sports injuries in children and young athletes, and none specifically addressing running injuries.[6] Currently, the youngest age group with reliable data is high school cross-country runners. Rauh and colleagues[7–9] have published several studies based on injury data collected from a large population of high school cross-country runners in Seattle, Washington, over a 15-year period. Injury data were collected using an injury surveillance system.

Department of Family Medicine, University of Virginia Health System, PO Box 800729, Charlottesville, VA 22908, USA
* Corresponding author.
E-mail address: cks2n@virginia.edu

Clin Sports Med 29 (2010) 499–511
doi:10.1016/j.csm.2010.03.005
sportsmed.theclinics.com

The study reported on injury rates, sites of injury, severity of injury, and gender and allowed for the comparison of injury rates in cross-country with other sports. The following summarizes the investigators' findings: (1) Cross-country running had a high rate of injuries compared with other high school sports. (2) Compared with boys, girls had a higher rate of injury and were more likely to sustain an injury that resulted in greater disability during the season. (3) The most common site of injury was the shin in girls and the knee in boys. (4) Once runners were injured, they had a 4- to 5-fold likelihood of reinjury at the same site.[6,7] Other studies have found that the female gender and runners with excessive quadriceps angles (Q-angles) were at a higher risk of injury during the season.[8,9] Plisky and colleagues[10] found that higher body mass indexes (BMIs) were associated with the development of medial tibial stress syndrome (MTSS). Data from these studies are the basis for future investigations in the young athletic population and underscore the importance of such work. Unfortunately, there are currently no such studies characterizing injuries in younger-aged running athletes.[6,11]

UNIQUE FEATURES OF THE GROWING ATHLETE

Because of the effects of growth on the musculoskeletal system, skeletally immature athletes are at higher risk for sustaining injuries at the tendon attachment sites (apophyses), joint surfaces (articular cartilage), and the growth plate (physis).[6,11] This article reviews the characteristics of the musculoskeletal system in the growing athlete and how these place them at risk for unique overuse injuries. The article also reviews the evaluation and treatment of these unique injuries as well as other injuries commonly seen in the young running athlete and concludes with a discussion on strategies to help prevent overtraining and overuse injuries in young athletes.

APOPHYSEAL DISORDERS

Apophyseal injuries are unique to the growing athlete and most commonly caused by overtraining. The apophysis is the insertion site of a tendon to the cartilage in growing bone. At this junction, a growth plate or secondary ossification center develops. Until the apophyses fuse at skeletal maturity, the connection between the apophysis and the underlying bone is weaker than the associated tendon or muscle. As a result, children and adolescents injure or inflame the apophysis (apophysitis) rather than the tendon (tendonitis) or muscle (strain) with overuse.[1–4,11] Because children's bones often grow at a faster rate than the adjacent muscles and tendons, muscle tightness and inflexibility may occur after a growth spurt. The increase in traction forces across the apophysis during this time seems to predispose to injury (traction apophysitis). Common sites of injury in the young runner include the heel (Sever disease), the knee (Osgood-Schlatter disease [OSD]), and the pelvis (pelvic apophysitis and apophyseal avulsion injury).[1–4,11]

Sever Disease

Calcaneal apophysitis, or Sever disease, is a traction apophysitis at the insertion of the Achilles tendon on the posterior calcaneus. It is the second most common apophyseal disorder, representing 8% of all overuse injuries in adolescent athletes.[12,13] Sever disease is more commonly seen in boys aged 10 to 12 years; it also occurs in girls aged 8 to 10 years. Children with high-arched (cavus) feet and tight Achilles tendons may be predisposed to calcaneal apophysitis.[12,14]

History

The classic presentation of Sever disease is a young athlete involved in a running or jumping sport, usually soccer or gymnastics, presenting with pain at the back and sides of the heel. The pain is often bilateral and usually occurs at the beginning of a new season or sport. Symptoms of the disease are exacerbated by activities such as running or jumping and relieved with rest.[13–15]

Examination

On inspection of an affected heel, mild swelling at the Achilles insertion site may be present. Direct palpation of the Achilles tendon is tender and ankle dorsiflexion is limited and painful. Pain may also be elicited with lateral compression of the posterior calcaneus. Diagnosis is based on clinical findings, the hallmark of which is restricted dorsiflexion and a positive squeeze test tenderness upon squeezing the lateral and medial calcaneus.[15]

Imaging

Radiographic imaging is not usually necessary but may help with the diagnosis of atypical cases. If indicated, a lateral view of the ankle proves most valuable because it shows the calcaneal growth plate. Findings may include increased sclerosis and fragmentation of the calcaneal apophysis; however, these findings are not specific and are also found in asymptomatic patients.[2,4,13,14] A comparison view of the asymptomatic ankle may be helpful.

Treatment

Treatment is conservative with a period of relative rest, during which time running and aggravating activities should be avoided. Ice massage, nonsteroidal antiinflammatory drugs (NSAIDs), or acetaminophen can be used for pain. As symptoms improve, low-impact exercises such as stationary biking, aquajogging, or swimming can begin. Cushioned heel lifts lessen the strain on the Achilles tendon. An Achilles tendon stretching program should be instituted followed by strengthening exercises for the plantar and dorsiflexors of the ankle. A gradual return to higher-impact activities can be expected over 6 to 8 weeks. Permanent resolution occurs with closure of the growth plate. Corticosteroid injection and surgery are contraindicated.[2,4,13,14]

Osgood-Schlatter Disease

OSD is a traction apophysitis of the tibial tuberosity and a common cause of knee pain in young athletes. It is the most common apophyseal disorder representing 10% of all overuse syndromes in adolescents.[13] OSD is commonly seen in athletes involved in sports requiring repetitive running, jumping, and cutting (quick turns), such as basketball, football, and soccer. It commonly occurs around a growth spurt in girls aged 12 to 14 years and boys aged 14 to 16 years.[2,4,16,17]

History

The athlete presents with knee pain and swelling over the tibial tubercle. Pain is often bilateral and aggravated by activities that require significant contraction of the quadriceps muscle, such as running, jumping, and squatting.[16,17]

Examination

Examination demonstrates tenderness and swelling over the tibial tuberosity. Pain can be reproduced with extension of the knee against resistance. Tightness of the quadriceps and hamstring muscles are also common findings.[16] Occasionally there is bony irregularity over the tubercle, which may appear enlarged from soft tissue swelling and fragmentation of the tubercle. The diagnosis is made clinically.[17]

Imaging

Radiographs are usually not required but can be helpful in refractory cases to rule out an avulsion fracture of the tibial tubercle.[18] A lateral view is most helpful to outline the tibial tubercle and profile the extensor mechanism. The lateral view may show separation of apophyses with fragmentation of the tibial tubercle and soft tissue swelling anterior to the tuberosity.[16,18]

Treatment

Treatment consists of rest, activity modification, and ice massage to reduce pain and swelling. NSAIDs or acetaminophen may be used for pain control in more severe cases. Low-impact aerobic exercises such as stationary biking, swimming, or aqua-jogging can assist with maintaining aerobic fitness while recovering. A stretching program should be instituted, targeting the quadriceps and hamstring muscles. Applying moist compresses to the tibial tubercle 15 minutes before activity followed by ice massage for 20 minutes after activity maybe helpful. Contact sports may require the use of a kneepad to protect the tender tibial tubercle.[16,18] The use of an infrapatellar strap for 6 to 8 weeks may provide symptomatic relief during activity. Corticosteroid injection of the tibial tubercle is not recommended. Symptoms typically improve over 4 to 6 weeks, with complete resolution in 12 to 18 months at the time of fusion of the tibial tubercle.[17,18] Occasionally, a nonunited fragment of bone develops at the site and requires surgical excision to relieve symptoms; otherwise, surgery is not indicated. Long-term sequelae include prominence of the tibial tubercle, which can cause pain on kneeling.[16–18]

Sinding-Larsen-Johansson Disease

Sinding-Larsen-Johansson disease is similar to OSD in that it is secondary to the pull of the quadriceps extensor mechanism on the apophysis. Anterior knee pain is believed to result from persistent traction at the immature inferior pole of the patella, leading to calcification and ossification at this junction. It usually affects active preteen boys between the ages of 10 and 12 years. Anterior knee pain is usually activity-related, especially with jumping, running, kneeling, or climbing stairs. The pain and swelling are usually localized at the inferior pole of the patella and are usually mild in severity and can be acute or chronic in duration. Point tenderness can be noted at the inferior pole of the patella and can sometimes be accentuated by resistance to quadriceps contraction. The remainder of the knee examination is usually normal. Plain radiographs are not needed for diagnosis.

Treatment is conservative and similar to OSD and almost always resolves without sequelae.[16,19]

APOPHYSEAL DISORDERS OF THE PELVIS

Apophyseal injuries of the pelvis are most commonly caused by sport participation and running. These injuries range from irritation of the apophysis (apophysitis) due to overuse to the acute apophyseal avulsion fracture that presents as an acute injury. Most apophyseal injuries resolve with conservative treatment.[20–22]

Pelvic Apophysitis

Pelvic apophysitis is an overuse injury that typically occurs because of repetitive overuse of the hip flexor muscles. The most commonly involved muscles are the sartorius and the rectus femoris, which attach at the anterior superior iliac spine (ASIS) and the anterior inferior iliac spine (AIIS), respectively. Adolescents with excessively tight hip and thigh muscles appear to be more prone to pelvis or hip apophysitis.[20]

History
The patient usually presents with the complaint of a gradual, dull activity-related pain located near the front or side of the hip. The discomfort is generally worsened by activity and relieved with rest. Distance runners are commonly affected secondary to the chronic repetitive tensile stress placed over the apophyseal areas.[20]

Examination
Pain can be reproduced with palpation of the affected pelvic apophysis (ASIS or AIIS) or with resisted hip flexion. Passive stretching of the hip flexor muscles also causes discomfort. The gait and passive range of motion of the hips are usually normal.[20]

Imaging
Radiographic evaluation may show widening of the apophysis but is often normal. In patients with severe symptoms, radiographs are mandatory to rule out an apophyseal avulsion fracture or other more severe hip conditions, such as slipped capital femoral epiphysis or Legg-Calvé-Perthes disease.[20–22]

Treatment
Treatment involves rest, applying ice to the affected area, and gradual functional rehabilitation. When daily activities can be tolerated without pain, gentle stretching and strengthening of the muscles that attach to the affected apophysis (the hip flexors and abdominal muscles) can begin. Once flexibility and strength have improved, sport-specific activities such as jogging can begin with gradual progress to full activity.[20–22]

Apophyseal Avulsion Injuries of the Pelvis

Pelvic avulsion injuries are seen in athletes participating in sports that require quick, explosive movements, such as track (sprinters and hurdlers), soccer, football, basketball, and gymnastics. The most common avulsion fractures occur at the ischial tuberosity where the hamstring muscles attach, followed by the AIIS and the ASIS, where the rectus femoris and sartorius muscles attach, respectively.[20] The mechanism of injury is a forceful contraction of the involved muscle group against the apophyseal attachment, resulting in separation of the apophysis from the body of the pelvis. This injury occurs more commonly in adolescent boys. Less common areas of avulsion are the iliac crest and the greater and lesser trochanters.[20–22]

History
The typical history involves the sudden onset of sharp pain in a young athlete in the buttock or anterior lateral hip while sprinting, jumping, or kicking. The pain is associated with an audible snap or pop and is usually severe enough that athletes are unable to continue their activity.[23] Many are unable to ambulate comfortably secondary to pain that is exacerbated by passive stretching of the involved muscle.[20,21]

Examination
On examination, the patient has an antalgic gait along with tenderness and swelling over the injured apophysis (ischial tuberosity, ASIS, or AIIS). Pain can be reproduced with passive stretching or active contraction of the affected muscle group. The passive range of motion of the hip joint is usually normal. Any limitation of passive hip flexion or internal rotation should raise suspicion for other hip joint pathology such as a slipped capital femoral epiphysis.[20,21,23]

Imaging

Radiographs should always be performed in young athletes with acute onset of hip or pelvic pain. An anteroposterior (AP) pelvis radiograph is usually adequate and allows a comparison view of the unaffected side. It is important to determine the size of the avulsed fragment (if any) and the degree of bone displacement. Radiographs also rule out other significant bony abnormalities such as fractures or epiphyseal injuries. Orthopedic referral is recommended for avulsion injuries with more than 2 cm of displacement.[20,21,23]

Treatment

Treatment includes relative rest and pain control measures with ice, NSAIDs, or acet-aminophen. Short-term use of crutches may be required, but limiting running and jumping is usually sufficient to control symptoms. When ambulation is pain free, a stretching and strengthening program can be instituted along with low-impact aerobic exercises. Progression is slowly made back to jogging, running, cutting, and jumping, with return to sports participation once full strength and pain-free range of motion is achieved. Anticipate 4 to 12 weeks for recovery and return to sport depending on the site of avulsion. Ischial tuberosity avulsions tend to be more severe than other avulsion injuries and frequently require 9 to 12 weeks for recovery. Patients not improving with conservative care may require orthopedic evaluation for surgical options.[20,21,23]

OSTEOCHONDRITIS DISSECANS OF THE KNEE

The immature articular cartilage on the joint surface in a young growing athlete is more susceptible to injury caused by shear forces than in adults.[4] Juvenile osteochondritis dissecans (OCD) of the knee is a disorder of the ossification centers in femoral sub-chondral bone, which results in the loss of support of the overlying articular cartilage followed by breakdown and fragmentation of the cartilage and bone.[19] The cause for this condition is unclear but is often attributed to repetitive axial loading and micro-trauma that occurs from intense physical activity. It is 3 times more common in boys than in girls, with the maximum incidence between the ages of 10 and 20 years. Most OCD lesions are found in the classic area of the posterolateral aspect of the medial femoral condyle.[24]

History

Young patients typically present with poorly localized knee pain that is exacerbated by exercise, particularly when climbing hills or stairs. Patients with stable lesions complain of knee pain and stiffness during or after activities, along with occasional swelling. In the later stages, patients complain of mechanical symptoms such as grinding, locking, and catching, secondary to loose or detached osteochondrotic lesions.[24–26]

Examination

In early stages, the examination shows tenderness over the anteromedial aspect of the knee, with varying amounts of knee flexion. This finding corresponds to the most common site of OCD lesions, the lateral aspect of the medial femoral condyle. Later in the course, patients develop evidence of quadriceps atrophy, decreased range of motion, and an effusion. The patient may begin to walk with an altered gait and externally rotate the affected leg to prevent pain. Unstable lesions are distingui-shable by the presence of mechanical symptoms, knee effusion, and pain with motion.[24,25]

Imaging

Evaluation should include plain radiography followed by magnetic resonance imaging (MRI). Initial radiographs should include AP, lateral, tunnel, and skyline views. Comparison views of the contralateral knee should be obtained to prevent confusion with normal bone development. The classic OCD lesion of the medial femoral condyle is best seen on the tunnel view and may not be apparent on AP radiographs. Although helpful, plain radiographs are poor at establishing the stability of the lesion or the state of the overlying cartilage. MRI is considered the gold standard for the evaluation of OCD. It provides information regarding the size, location, staging, and progression or healing of the lesion.[24,25]

Treatment

Treatment may be conservative or operative depending on several factors, including the age of the patient, the fragment size, location, and stability. Nonoperative treatment may be considered in young patients with open physes and a stable lesion on MRI. Several studies have demonstrated successful healing (>90% of patients) using a conservative treatment regimen in these patients. The treatment requires a non–weight-bearing status with knee immobilization and daily range of motion exercises for 6 weeks followed by pain-free activity modification over 3 to 6 months. Patients who do not improve with conservative management over 6 to 12 months should be referred for operative management.[24,25] Patients with closed physes or those approaching skeletal maturity should be treated more aggressively. The success of conservative management for these patients is much lower. Therefore, these patients and any patient with an unstable lesion should be referred for surgical intervention.[24,25]

RUNNING INJURIES COMMON TO ALL AGE GROUPS
Patellofemoral Syndrome

Patellofemoral syndrome (PFS) is one of the most common causes of anterior knee pain in young runners, with females more commonly affected.[1] The onset of symptoms frequently follows a change in training, such as an increase in mileage or intensity of training. The cause is multifactorial and includes overuse, poor patellar tracking, trauma, and malalignment of the lower extremity or extensor mechanism. Runners who have increased internal rotation of the hip, external rotation of the lower leg, knock-knee alignment, flat feet, tight hamstrings, and poor quadriceps muscle tone are also at increased risk.[27,28]

History
Patients often present with anterior knee pain in one or both knees, which becomes worse with running, squatting, or when ascending and descending stairs.[1] The pain can be retropatellar, peripatellar, or diffuse and described as aching but can also become sharp and burning.[19] Frequently, there is pain with prolonged sitting ("theater sign"), and patients report the need to straighten their legs out to decrease discomfort.[4,29]

Examination
The knee examination reveals nonspecific peripatellar tenderness and pain with patellar compression. The quadriceps may show weakness or decreased tone especially in the vastus medialis obliquus muscle group. The hamstring muscles may also demonstrate inflexibility.[1] Examination of the lower extremity and foot may reveal other risk factors associated with PFS, such as angular or rotational deformities and high arches (pes cavus) or flat feet (pes planus).[29]

Imaging

PFS is usually a clinical diagnosis and imaging is unnecessary initially. However, imaging is indicated in patients who fail to improve within 4 to 6 weeks of conservative therapy.

Treatment

Treatment is conservative with the main goals of reducing pain, improving patellar tracking and alignment, and returning the patient to as high a level of function as possible. Pain is controlled initially with ice massage, rest, and activity modification. Short-term use of NSAIDs or acetaminophen can also be used. Once pain is controlled, the patient may begin a structured rehabilitation program focusing on quadriceps and core muscle strengthening and hamstring flexibility. Patellar bracing and taping can decrease pain and improve function in a subgroup of individuals. Orthotics can be beneficial for those who have excessive foot pronation. As symptoms improve, a slow graduated return to activities may commence with particular attention paid to correcting previous training errors.[1,4,19,26]

Shin Splints/MTSS

MTSS is a condition seen in runners that results in pain and discomfort in the posteromedial aspect of the distal two-thirds of the tibia. The condition is caused by overtraining and can occur in running athletes who train on hard surfaces, have poor footwear, or recently increased their training intensity or mileage.[1,30] MTSS is common in cross-country runners and seems to affect women more than men. Biomechanical abnormalities such as pes planus or cavus, tarsal coalition, leg length discrepancies, and muscular imbalances may also contribute. Additional risk factors include excessive foot pronation and higher BMI.[31]

History

Patients complain of a dull ache along the posteromedial portion of the distal tibia, which is made worse with running and gets better with rest.[31] The pain continues to progress if training is not decreased, and performance is eventually affected. More severe cases can have pain with activities of daily living.[31]

Examination

Palpation over the medial tibia demonstrates diffuse, nonfocal tenderness.[31] Rarely, there may be some mild swelling noted over the distal portion of the tibia.[30] Pain may be reproduced with resisted plantar flexion or toe raises. Differentiation between MTSS and a stress fracture can be difficult. MTSS symptoms are usually more diffuse along the tibia, whereas a stress fracture produces more localized pain.[31]

Imaging

Plain radiographs are usually normal and of little utility initially. The diagnosis should be made clinically. For patients with persistent symptoms or concerns of a stress fracture, an MRI or bone scan should be obtained to clarify the diagnosis.[31]

Treatment

Treatment for MTSS includes relative rest with avoidance of exacerbating activities such as running on hard surfaces or hill training. Ice massage, NSAIDs, or acetaminophen may be used to control inflammation and pain. Nonimpact cross-training exercise with an elliptical machine, stationary bike, swimming, or aquajogging can assist with maintaining aerobic fitness. Biomechanical factors should be identified and addressed, and a course of physical therapy prescribed to improve lower extremity strength and flexibility. Orthotics may be helpful for patients with foot hyperpronation.

Most patients respond to these conservative measures and slowly return to physical activity.[30,31]

Stress Fractures

Stress fractures are a common overuse injury in runners and usually occur in the lower extremity because of excessive, repetitive loading of the weight-bearing bones. These fractures commonly involve the lower third of the tibia but can also occur in the metatarsals, tarsal bones, femur, and the fibula. The cause is multifactorial, but common risk factors include a sudden increase in volume or intensity of physical activity, history of previous stress fracture, hard running surface, poor footwear, overtraining, and the female gender, especially if there is a history of menstrual or eating disorder and osteoporosis.[1,30]

When there is a sudden increase in the running regimen, an excessive stress is applied to the bones of the lower extremity, producing an imbalance between bone resorption and bone formation. This imbalance leads to weakening of the bone and the development of microfractures and, with continued loading, the development of a stress fracture.[2,32,33] Stress fractures in runners can be classified as low- and high-risk based on the potential for complications such as nonunion and progression to complete fracture. Low-risk sites include posteromedial tibia, metatarsal shafts (second to fourth), sacrum, and pubic rami. High-risk sites include femoral head, superior side of the femoral neck (tension side), anterior cortex of the tibia (tension side), tarsal navicular, patella, medial malleolus, talus, proximal fifth metatarsal, sesamoids (great toe), and base of the second metatarsal bone.[33–35]

History

The runner complains of the gradual onset of vague pain localized to the involved bone or area that increases with increased activity or running. With continued training, the pain progresses and becomes present with less strenuous activity and eventually persists even at rest. Pain of a stress fracture is local, sharp, and exacerbated by weight-bearing activity. Symptoms typically follow a change in training activity such as an increase in running mileage or pace, hill running, or running on hard surfaces. Patients with tibial stress fractures may have had a previous diagnosis of shins splints or MTSS.[1,30,33]

Examination

Examination demonstrates localized tenderness over the involved bone with occasional overlying swelling or a palpable callus. Patients with tibial stress fractures have reproducible pain with jumping up and down on the involved leg (the hop test). The hop test should not be performed in patients suspected of having stress fractures of the femoral neck because of risk of complete fracture.[1,30,33]

Imaging

The diagnosis of a stress fracture is often made by analyzing the patient's history and by physical examination. Plain radiographs are usually normal for the first 2 to 3 weeks of symptoms. Positive findings include periosteal elevation, cortical thickening, sclerosis, or a true fracture line. Traditionally, nuclear bone scan was used to diagnose stress fractures, but more recently MRI has become the study of choice. MRI has been shown to be highly sensitive and specific for diagnosing stress fractures and should be used when there is a need for a definitive diagnosis.[1,30,33]

Treatment

Management of the fractures depends on the fracture location and the risk for complications. Pain control is managed with ice and crutches (if weight bearing causes pain). NSAIDs are not recommended because of evidence that they may interfere with healing. Acetaminophen or tramadol may also be used if additional pain control is required.[36,37] Low-risk stress fractures are treated with avoidance of activities that cause pain until healing has occurred. For low-risk stress fractures, the athlete should modify activity to include complete rest for 1 month during which cross-training with aquajogging (deep water running) or stationary biking is allowed, if pain free. In tibial stress fractures, bracing with a long-leg pneumatic stirrup splint may decrease the time required to return to full activity.[33] A walking boot may be used for the patient with metatarsal stress fractures. A gradual return to weight-bearing activities is allowed when the runner is pain-free, which may take 4 to 6 weeks. Runners may then start on a graduated walking and jogging program for 8 to 10 weeks with slow weekly progression as long as they remain pain free. It is recommended to increase the total weekly training regimen (either time or distance) by no more than 10% per week. Return to full-time running may take anywhere from 2 to 4 months.[1,30,34] Physical therapy can help identify and address biomechanical risk factors. Runners with foot hyperpronation may benefit from the use of orthotics. Training errors should also be addressed, including the choice and maintenance of appropriate running shoes.[1,30]

High-risk stress fractures may require prolonged rest and immobilization. In cases of delayed union or nonunion, orthopedic consultation may be needed. Special caution should be given to patients with a suspected stress fracture of the femoral head or neck. Stress fractures involving the superior aspect of the femoral neck (tension side) are at high risk of complete fracture. These patients should be made non–weight bearing until imaging can be obtained to clarify the diagnosis.[35]

MARATHON RUNNING IN CHILDREN

There are many young runners who have trained and completed a full 26.2-mile marathon race. This raises the question, "how much athletic training is too much?" Unfortunately, there are no scientifically determined guidelines to help define how much exercise is healthy and beneficial to the young athlete versus what might be harmful and represent overtraining.[3] In 2003, the American Academy of Pediatrics (AAP) Council on Sports Medicine and Fitness published a position statement regarding the participation of children (<18 years of age) in marathon running. In the position statement, the AAP strongly recommended against marathon running in young runners citing concerns for overuse injuries and possible psychological burn out due to the rigors of training.[38] However, their recommendations lacked the support of scientific data and were challenged by other investigators.[39] Thus, in 2007 the AAP revised their position on marathon running, acknowledging the lack of evidence to support or refute the safety of children participating in marathon running. In their revised statement, the AAP recommended a well-designed weekly training program that ensured safe running conditions and provided appropriate education on endurance training. They also strongly recommended that special consideration be given to environmental heat stress and appropriate hydration guidelines as young runners are at increased risk for heat injury compared with adults.[3] The AAP referred to its previous position statement on this subject published in 2000, which provided guidelines for preventing heat injury in young athletes.[40] The AAP felt that as long as there is a well-designed training program in place, there is no reason to disallow the participation of a young athlete in a properly run marathon, provided the athlete is enjoying the activity and is without injury.[3] The ideal training program would allow young runners to train at distances appropriate for their development and ability. Coaches and trainers of young runners should keep the runners' overall health at the forefront of priorities. Running regimens, surfaces, shoes, techniques, and conditioning programs should be chosen to protect the child and minimize injuries.[6]

OVERTRAINING AND BURNOUT IN YOUNG ATHLETES

In recent years, more and more athletes are undertaking intense training regimens at younger ages, thereby increasing their risk for overuse injuries and possible burnout.[3,5] In the pursuit of an Olympic dream or college scholarship, many young athletes are specializing in a single sport, beginning at a very young age with year-round training and competition.[3] The ever-increasing requirements to be successful at a highly competitive level create a constant pressure for athletes to train longer and harder.[41] The AAP has noted that these athletes are at a higher risk of overtraining injuries and burnout. Unfortunately, there are few studies to help guide clinicians and trainers regarding the appropriate amount of training recommended to avoid overtraining and overuse injuries.[41]

Burnout, or overtraining syndrome, has been well described in the literature for adult athletes involved in endurance sports but has not been reported in the younger athlete. The burnout syndrome is thought to be caused by a series of psychological, physiologic, and hormonal changes that result in decreased sports performance. Manifestations include chronic muscle or joint pain, personality changes, elevated resting heart rate, and decreased sports performance. Young athletes may have fatigue, lack of enthusiasm about practice or competition, or difficulty in successfully completing usual routines.[3,41,42]

The AAP Council on Sports Medicine and Fitness addressed these concerns by publishing guidelines for preventing overtraining, overuse injuries, and burnout in young athletes.[3] The guidelines were to assist clinicians caring for young athletes involved in intense year-round training. The AAP recommended the encouragement of a well-rounded, multisport athlete stating that the athletes have the best chance of achieving the goal of lifelong fitness and enjoyment of physical activity. The AAP voiced concern regarding the trend of young athletes specializing in a single sport with year-round training and competition. The AAP reminded clinicians that the ultimate goal of sports participation was to promote lifelong physical activity, recreation, and skills of healthy competition that are useful in all aspects of life.[3] To that end the AAP recommended the following guidelines for preventing overtraining, overuse injuries, and burnout in young athletes: (1) Encourage athletes to take at least 1 to 2 days off from athletic training each week. (2) Advise athletes to not increase their weekly training regimen by more than 10% per week. (3) Recommend that athletes take 2 to 3 months off from a specific sport each year to allow for physical and mental recovery, and to work on strength and conditioning. (4) Emphasize that sports participation should be for fun, sportsmanship, safety, and skill acquisition. (5) Be alert to signs and symptoms of burnout or overtraining, including nonspecific muscle or joint problems, fatigue, or poor academic performance.[3]

FUTURE RESEARCH NEEDED

Unfortunately, the current recommendations for training and injury prevention in childhood athletes are predominantly based on committee consensus and expert opinion. There are no substantial scientific data available to rely on. The literature is currently lacking in regard to the study of overuse injuries in young athletes and runners. Furthermore, there have been no preventive trials that have focused specifically on measures to reduce the risk for overuse injuries in young children and adolescent athletes.[6] This lack of data underscores the importance of establishing large-scale injury surveillance systems that can provide reliable data on injury trends in sports, including running for boys and girls. Accurate and descriptive injury data allow for the identification and testing of risk factors and preventive measures in preventing overuse injuries,[6] an area of study that is ripe for further investigation. Future studies will pave the way for evidence-based guidelines to assist physicians, athletic trainers, and coaches in setting up training and prevention strategies to make athletic activities safer and more enjoyable for young athletes.

REFERENCES

1. Soprano JV, Fuchs SM. Common overuse injuries in the pediatric and adolescent athlete. Clin Pediatr Emerg Med 2007;8:7–14.
2. Cassas KJ, Cassettari-Wayhs A. Childhood and adolescent sports-related overuse injuries. Am Fam Physician 2006;73:1014–22.
3. Brenner JS, The Council on Sports Medicine and Fitness. Overuse injuries, overtraining, and burnout in child and adolescent athletes. Clinical report. Pediatrics 2007;119:1242–5.
4. Adirim TA, Cheng TL. Overview of injuries in the young athlete. Sports Med 2003; 33(1):75–81.
5. National Federation of High Schools survey of participation. Available at: http://www.nfhs.org/Participation/. Accessed November 17, 2009.
6. Caine D, Maffulli N, Caine C. Epidemiology of injury in child and adolsecent sports: injury rates, risk factors, and prevention. Clin Sports Med 2008;27:19–50.
7. Rauh MJ, Margherita AJ, Rice SG, et al. High school cross country running injuries: a longitudinal study. Clin J Sport Med 2000;10:110–6.
8. Rauh MJ, Koepsell TD, Rivara FP, et al. Epidemiology of musculoskeletal injuries among high school cross-country runners. Am J Epidemiol 2006;163:151–9.
9. Rauh MJ, Koepsell TD, Vivar FP, et al. Quadriceps angle and risk of injury among high school cross-country runners. J Orthop Sports Phys Ther 2007;37(12): 725–33.
10. Plisky MS, Rauh MJ, Geiderscheit B, et al. Medial tibial stress syndrome in high school cross-country runners: incidence and risk factors. J Orthop Sports Phys Ther 2007;37(2):40–7.
11. Logsdon VK. Training the prepubertal and pubertal athlete. Curr Sports Med Rep 2007;6:183–9.
12. Rockwell PG. Adolescents sports injuries and the preparticipation physical evaluation. Clin Fam Pract 2000;2(4):837–62.
13. Maffulli N, Wong J, Almekinders LC. Types and epidemiology of tendinopathy. Clin Sports Med 2003;22:675–92.
14. Madden CC, Mellion MB. Sever's disease and other causes of heel pain in adolescents. Am Fam Physician 1996;54(6):1995–2000.
15. Kennedy JG, Knowles B, Dolan M, et al. Foot and ankle injuries in the adolescent runner. Curr Opin Pediatr 2005;17:34–42.
16. Gholve PA, Scher DM, Khakharia S, et al. Osgood Schlatter syndrome. Curr Opin Pediatr 2007;19(1):44–50.
17. Martin TJ, Martin JS. Special issues and concerns for the high school- and college-aged athletes. Pediatr Clin North Am 2002;49(3):533–52.

18. Duri ZA, Patel DV, Aichroth PM. The immature athlete. Clin Sports Med 2002; 21(3):461–82.
19. Frank JB, Jarit GJ, Brayman JT, et al. Lower extremity injuries in the skeletally immature athlete. J Am Acad Orthop Surg 2007;15:356–66.
20. Moeller JL. Pelvic and hip apophyseal avulsion injuries in young athletes. Curr Sports Med Rep 2003;2(2):110–5.
21. Kocher MS, Rucker R. Pediatric athlete hip disorders. Clin Sports Med 2006;25: 211–53.
22. Adkins SB, Figler RA. Hip pain in athletes. Am Fam Physician 2000;61(7): 2109–18.
23. Anderson SJ. In: Sports injuries, current problems in pediatric and adolescent health care, 35. St Louis (MO): Elsevier Inc; 2005. 110–64.
24. Robertson W, Kelly B, Green D. Osteochondritis dissecans of the knee in children. Curr Opin Pediatr 2003;15:38–44.
25. Kocher M, Tucker R, Ganley TJ, et al. Management of osteochondritis dissecans of the knee. Am J Sports Med 2006;34(7):1181–91.
26. Kaeding CC, Whitehead R. Musculoskeletal injuries in adolescents. Prim Care 1998;25(1):211–23.
27. Ganley TJ, Gaugles RL, Moroz LA. Consultation with the specialist: patellofemoral conditions in childhood. Pediatr Rev 2006;27:264–70.
28. Thomee R, Augustsson J, Karisson J. Patellofemoral pain syndrome: a review of current issues. Sports Med 1999;28:245.
29. Post WR. Clinical evaluation of patients with patellofemoral disorders. Arthroscopy 1999;15:841.
30. Pell RF 4th, Khanuja HS, Cooley GR. Leg pain in the running athlete. J Am Acad Orthop Surg 2004;12(6):396–404.
31. Moen MH, Tol JL, Weir A, et al. Medial tibial stress syndrome: a critical review. Sports Med 2009;39(7):523–46.
32. Heyworth BE, Green DW. Lower extremity stress fractures in pediatric and adolescent athletes. Curr Opin Pediatr 2008;20:58–61.
33. Lassus J, Tulikoura I, Konttinen YT, et al. Bone stress injuries of the lower extremity: a review. Acta Orthop Scand 2002;73(3):359–68.
34. Boden BP, Osbahr DC, Jimenez C. Low-risk stress fractures. Am J Sports Med 2001;29:100.
35. Boden BP, Osbahr DC. High-risk stress fractures: evaluation and treatment. J Am Acad Orthop Surg 2000;8:344.
36. Wheeler P, Batt ME. Do non-steroidal anti-inflammatory drugs adversely affect stress fracture healing? A short review. Br J Sports Med 2005;39:65.
37. Stovitz SD, Arendt EA. NSAIDs should not be used in treatment of stress fractures. Am Fam Physician 2004;70:1452.
38. Rice SG, Waniewski S. Children and marathoning: how young is too young? Clin J Sport Med 2003;13:369–73.
39. Roberts WO. Children and running: at what distance safe? [Letter to the Editor]. Clin J Sport Med 2005;15(2):109–10.
40. Anderson SJ, The Committee on Sports Medicine and Fitness. Climatic heat stress and the exercising child and adolescent. Pediatrics 2000;106(1):158–9.
41. American Academy of Pediatrics Committee on Sports Medicine and Fitness. Intensive training and sports specialization in young athletes. Pediatrics 2000; 106:154–7.
42. Small E. Chronic musculoskeletal pain in young athletes. Pediatr Clin North Am 2002;49:655–62.

Index

Note: Page numbers of article titles are in **boldface** type.

A

Amenorrhea, in female runners, 486
Ankle, joint kinetics at, factors influencing, 357
Apophyseal avulsion injuries, of pelvis, 503–504
Apophyseal disorders, in pediatric athlete, 500–502
Apophysitis, pelvic, 502–503
Arm movement, as source of propulsion in distance running, 360
Athletic performance, flexibility training and, 369

B

Bony abnormalities, patellar malalignment and instability in, 379–381
Braces, patellar, in patellofemoral pain, 393

C

Calcaneal apophysitis, 500–501
Cardiovascular dysfunction, in female runners, 487
Center of pressure, on foot, 354, 355
    origin of, 357
    rise and fall of, 357–358
Children, marathon running by, 508–509
Collapsed Athlete Algorithm, 464, 465

E

Endothelial dysfunction, in female runners, 487–488
Entrapment neuropathies, diagnosis and management of, 437
    in runners, 437–457
Exertional collapse, clinical findings, ECG findings, and evaluation of conditions in, 469, 470
    conditions associated with, 459–460
    diagnostic testing in, 472–473
    epidemiology of, 460–461, 462
    exercise-associated, 460, 461–462
        algorithm for approach to, 466, 467
    exercise-related, 460
        algorithm for approach to, 471
        differential diagnosis of, 463
        fieldside management of, 463–468
        patient responsiveness in, 464, 465
    in runners, evaluation and management of, **459–476**
    office-based management of, 468–471
    outpatient consultation/treatment following, 473

Clin Sports Med 29 (2010) 513–519
doi:10.1016/S0278-5919(10)00036-0
0278-5919/10/$ – see front matter © 2010 Elsevier Inc. All rights reserved.

sportsmed.theclinics.com

Moving?

Make sure your subscription moves with you!

To notify us of your new address, find your **Clinics Account Number** (located on your mailing label above your name), and contact customer service at:

Email: **journalscustomerservice-usa@elsevier.com**

800-654-2452 (subscribers in the U.S. & Canada)
314-447-8871 (subscribers outside of the U.S. & Canada)

Fax number: **314-447-8029**

Elsevier Health Sciences Division
Subscription Customer Service
3251 Riverport Lane
Maryland Heights, MO 63043

*To ensure uninterrupted delivery of your subscription, please notify us at least 4 weeks in advance of move.